Gertrude Poe

SLIM FOR HIM

SLIM FOR HIM

(Biblical Devotions On Diet)

by

PATRICIA BANTA KREML

Logos International
Plainfield, New Jersey

All Scripture is taken from the King
James Version except where noted
as TAB (The Amplified Bible).

Thanks . . .

To Chris Kreml, my husband. Thank you for putting up with me through the rough times and standing by me as a helper in all things. I love you.

To V.I.E.W. 1977. Thanks for being interested in the book and supporting me as I wrote (and typed some).

To Bill and Irene Banta for sharing their faith and their son, Billy, with me. All of these things have helped me to grow in the Lord to the point of writing this book.

To my family for loving me enough to give me the freedom to grow in faith in the direction I felt I should. I love you all.

To the radio ministry of Joan Cavanaugh, which helped me to face gluttony and fat and helped me to win the victory in Jesus.

To all those countless brothers and sisters who have supported me in love! Praise God!

Acknowledgments

The only acknowledgment is to the Father, Jesus Christ and the Holy Spirit as they are responsible for the writing of this book. Without the teaching of the Spirit, it could never have been written.

Introduction

The Lord is doing a mighty work, in the area of diet and eating habits, to set His people free by teaching them who they are in Him and what their rights and *responsibilities* are as His children. The book is meant to share some of these truths as well as set some basic guidelines for walking in His will concerning diet. Only God himself can give you a tailor-made plan of action, for only He can know your total needs. There are, however, some basic truths that apply to all and this book endeavors to present these with scriptural support.

Let the Spirit guide you and teach you those things God would have you to see. If at some point you can't agree with me, put that information on a shelf, accept what you can and go on. The Lord will lead you in His ways perfectly even as you seek Him. I pray that as you are blessed by what you read, you will share with other brothers and sisters who so desperately need this message of deliverance and healing.

Love,
In Jesus' Name

P.G.B. Kreml

P.G.B. Kreml

SLIM FOR HIM

Forbidden Fruit

And the Lord God commanded the man, saying, Of every tree of the garden thou mayest freely eat: But of the tree of the knowledge of good and evil, thou shalt not eat of it: for in the day that thou eatest thereof thou shalt surely die. (Gen. 2:16-17)

It is no coincidence that God should choose a rule concerning eating as the first and only commandment for Adam and Eve. From the moment of our conception, food is vitally important, for without nourishment we cannot live, and without proper nourishment we cannot grow strong and healthy. God did not make unreasonable requests of Adam and Eve concerning eating, neither does He do so of us. In their case, they could eat any food in the garden except of the tree of knowledge of good and evil. Why? Because it was the only "food" there that was harmful to them—both spiritually and physically harmful.

With us however, the list is longer and more complex, because man has created an abundance of harmful foods and has made even the physically harmless food a spiritual stumbling block. What are some of the "forbidden fruits" in your life?

Father, help me to see where I am missing you. Teach me concerning those things which are physically and spiritually harmful to me, not anyone else, just me. Show me my own personal "forbidden fruit." I ask this by faith, in Jesus' name, and I thank you in advance for the answer.

Appearances Are Deceiving

And when the woman saw that the tree was good for food, and that it was pleasant to the eyes, and a tree to be desired to make one wise, she took of the fruit thereof and gave also unto her husband with her; and he did eat. (Gen. 3:6)

From the beginning of time, man has always sought to be better than he was and, while improvement in itself is not wrong, man's efforts at improving himself have often gotten him into trouble. Eve saw that the food was good to eat, appetizing, and would change her life and make her someone she wanted to be. Does this apply to us today? Of course it does. Think of all the commercials we hear and see every day. Drink a certain sugary drink and you'll be slim, young, and beautiful just like the blonde on TV, and you'll have all the men running after you. Now that's Satan's lie to you, his sales job. Just as Adam and Eve got an unexpected result when they ate the forbidden fruit, so do we usually get the opposite of what we've been promised by the commercials. Instead of being slim, lively, and popular, we gain two pounds and hate ourselves in the morning. It is time for us to realize that the source of these lies is Satan. He's continuing an ongoing work which he began in the Garden of Eden. Are you going to continue to fall for his old line?

One other significant factor in this Scripture is, ". . . and gave also unto her husband with her; and he did eat." Isn't that just the way compulsive eaters are? We don't want to eat alone. We need company to make us feel we're really doing okay. Of course, we usually don't have to do much persuading. Adam was there, he heard the devil's pitch, and he knew better. But he saw Eve enjoying herself, and she obviously didn't drop dead. So he charged ahead and munched away. Think of all the times you've eaten food that was just junk and could only harm you, just because you saw skinny little Sally or Joe do it with no obvious ill effects. How did it affect you? That's right, you gained weight and felt awful.

Father, I don't want to follow the crowd into sin. Teach me to be wise in the foods I eat and the things I do. Lord, I know that you have made me intelligent enough to know that what looks good isn't always good for me. When you see me falling for a lie, remind me that it is not for me. Father, keep me also from tempting someone else.

Don't Pass the Buck

> And the man said, The woman whom thou gavest to be with me, she gave me of the tree, and I did eat. And the Lord God said unto the woman, What is this that thou hast done? And the woman said, The serpent beguiled me, and I did eat. (Gen. 3:12-13)

We now see that even in the beginning man learned quickly how to pass the buck. It's so hard for us to admit that we "ate the whole thing" that we try to excuse our own gluttony and sin by blaming someone else. Adam blamed Eve directly for giving him the fruit, and God indirectly for giving him Eve. But when it comes right down to it, he has to say, ". . . and *I* did eat." Eve blames the serpent, but also has to admit that she did the actual wrong by eating.

Just because mother sets a homemade lemon meringue pie in front of you doesn't mean you have to eat it. The sin comes when *you* pick up the fork and take that first mouthful. Mother may have been the tempter, but we are the ones who give in to the temptation. Why? Because we want to; we are greedy and our priorities are wrong. Why did Adam and Eve eat that fruit? Just because it was different and forbidden? No, they ate out of greed, a desire to be like God. They wanted to satisfy their own lust. Isn't that why the glutton eats—to satisfy his own craving?

What temptation will you face today? No matter what it is, you can resist it because God is more powerful than Satan.

When the temptation comes, simply say a firm no and add, "I'm going on with God." Then move on, don't argue your point and don't dwell on the offer. Claim the victory in Jesus' name.

Father, I know that you are all powerful and are able to help me out of any temptation. I also know that it is not your will that I should fall, and so I ask in Jesus' name that you sustain me in strength no matter what I may come up against. I know that through your strength I can be victorious, so teach me to reach for you, not the lemon pie, because you are sweeter by far and can surely satisfy all my desires.

Don't Look Back

But his wife looked back from behind him, and she became a pillar of salt. (Gen. 19:26)

Sodom and Gomorrah were two cities in which sin ran rampant, and the Lord had to destroy them. Some of the main sins were: adultery, fornication, homosexuality, drunkenness, and gluttony. The Lord remembered Lot and his family and sent angels to bring them out of the city before He destroyed it. Although God wished to spare Lot's whole family, his two sons-in-law refused to go and were left. Why did they choose to stay when they were told the city would be destroyed? For the same reasons gluttons and compulsive eaters continue in their sin: they love what they are doing and they don't believe destruction is just around the corner. Today, we tell ourselves, "I'll go on a diet after the holidays or the weekend." We always think we have time. Some of us do make it out before the heart attack or various diseases destroy our bodies, but many procrastinate too long. God is telling His people today, "Come out of your own personal Sodom and Gomorrah of gluttony. Let me save you from your own self-destruction."

"But what about Lot's wife?" you say. "She left like God said, and she still was destroyed." Yes, she was, but why? Because God told them not to look back, and she did. She knew God said she would be destroyed, but she looked back anyway. Was it just curiosity? No, she was looking back because that's where her true affections were.

Now God won't turn us into pillars of salt for looking back today; but by yearning for those things which are left behind, we say to Him, "I love these foods more than your perfect way of life. Even though they bring me fat and sickness and destruction, I still love them." Let's ask forgiveness for having done this and really repent. What is it that you've been looking back at? Leave it behind today and move on with the Lord.

Father, forgive me for looking back at those foods that tempt me. Lord, I want to go on with you, and I know you wouldn't ask me to give them up if it weren't for my own good. I sacrifice them to you as a love offering and I will no longer look back to them for pleasure and joy, but I will look ahead to you. Thank you, Father, for your forgiveness in Jesus' name.

Certain Priorities

> And there was set meat before him to eat: but he said, I will not eat, until I have told mine errand. And he said, Speak on. (Gen. 24:33)

The servant of Abraham had just come to the end of a long, hard journey in search of a wife for Abraham's son, Isaac. I'm sure the servant was exhausted and famished by the time he was finally in the home of Nehor and Milcah. The Scripture says food was set before him, but he refused to eat until he had fulfilled his purpose in coming—to seek Rebekah for Isaac. This is a fine example of a faithful servant as well as a man who has put food in its proper place.

To the compulsive eater, allowing one's self to get hungry is ridiculous, let alone delaying a meal for someone else. What would you have done in this servant's place? If God sent you out to perform a task for Him, would you have stopped to eat and then served the Lord? Your answer to that question (in all honesty) will give you some insight on where you are with God and what degree of importance food has in your life. If you would have eaten first, or don't really know what you would have done, chances are food still has too important a place in your life. We should eat to live, not live to eat.

This servant, I'm sure, enjoyed food as much as the next person, but he had his priorities in line. Do you want to be this kind of servant for God? You can begin today by asking God what your priorities really are and then asking what they should be. Truly the peace that comes from serving God first will far surpass the feeling of a full stomach and the hunger of an empty soul.

Father, please show me today where my priorities lie. Make me to face them in truth and see them as they are. Change them, Lord, and show me your perfect will for me in this area. I know in my mind that you must come first, but today I want that knowledge in my heart. Forgive me for putting you and your work second, and myself and food first. I thank you for forgiveness and by faith I receive the knowledge that you have given me concerning priorities. Thank you, loving Father.

Hunger vs. Appetite

Jacob was boiling pottage (lentil stew) one day, when Esau came from the field and was faint (with hunger). And Esau said to Jacob, I beg of you, let me have some of that red lentil stew to eat, for I am faint and famished! That is why his name was called Edom (red). Jacob answered, Then sell me today your birthright—the rights of a first-born. Esau said, See here, I am at the point of death; what good can this birthright do me? Jacob said, Swear to me today (that you are selling it to me), and he swore to Jacob and sold him his birthright. Then Jacob gave Esau bread and stew of lentils, and he ate and drank, and rose up and went his way. Thus Esau scorned his birthright as beneath his notice. (Gen. 25:29-34, TAB)

Jacob and Esau were twin brothers. Esau came out of his mother's womb first, so he had the right of the first-born. Now that doesn't have much significance today, but in his time it was extremely important. The first-born was entitled to the headship over his brothers, a double portion of his father's goods, and he succeeded his father as priest and ruler of his house. He was also entitled to his father's parting blessing. So you see it was not a light thing for Esau to sell his birthright. Why did he do it? Because he was tired and hungry, that's all. There is no indication that he was really starving to death. Many people have gone without food for more than forty days and did not die, so we know he was not at death's door. No, he sold the prized possession of his birthright to satisfy his impatience or his lust for food.

Most first-born men treasured their birthright, but compared to his lust for food when he was "hungry," Esau scorned his. Now you say, "I wouldn't have been that stupid!" Oh, yes, you would have, and *are*, and it isn't stupid, it's misguided. God gives us a healthy, strong, active body to enjoy His blessings of life and vitality, and we'll sell that daily for the pleasure of overindulging. We forfeit that peaceful, close communion with the Father because our desire for food is greater than our desire for His sincere, satisfying fellowship. How many times have we gone on a diet only to break it with the excuse, "Well, I missed lunch today and I just can't wait until dinner is ready. I'm starving! Let's go out to eat, and I'll go back on my diet tomorrow." It seems like a good enough excuse at the time, but later we have great remorse, just as Esau did.

When you're hungry today, do this for the Lord. Stop and ask yourself, "Am I really starving? Is this hunger really that bad? Can I really not wait to eat?" If you are really honest, I believe you'll make a remarkable discovery about yourself that will help you on your way to total freedom from compulsive and wrong eating.

Father, teach me to reverence your fellowship more than my love for food. Show me, Lord, the difference between "hunger" and "appetite." Forgive me for all the times I chose food over you and came out hungering in my soul and heart. I accept your forgiveness and thank you for it.

Only What's Needed

When they measured it with an omer, he who gathered much had nothing over, and he who gathered little had no lack; each gathered according to his need. Moses said, Let none of it be left until morning. But they did not listen to Moses; some of them left of it until morning, and it bred worms, became foul and stank; and Moses was angry with them. They gathered it every morning each as much as he needed; for when the sun became hot it melted. (Exod. 16:18-21, TAB)

Here we see God feeding the Israelites with manna in the desert. Each day the people would go out in the morning and gather manna for the day's food, according to the amount they needed. Note that God wanted them to have all the food they *needed* from Him each day and no one was to lack or overeat. But some were greedy and held extra back for the next day, even when they were told not to, and it rotted. God was teaching His people that He would be faithful each day to meet their need. Those who held back wanted more than their share. They knew God would send only as much as was needed, so they hoarded extra to meet their own desires. The result was Moses' and God's anger.

Are we guilty of such things today? Think about your favorite foods. Did you ever hide that last piece of cake so you could have it later? Do you ever find yourself hoping there will be leftovers from your favorite dish so you can eat it all by yourself the next day? Do you stuff yourself with your favorite foods when you have them because you're afraid you won't be able to have them again (especially if you're about to go on a diet)? All these are similar breaches of trust in God. It may be that God will take that favorite food away, but not unless you give it to Him first. Hoarding food and stuffing it in because you enjoy it isn't really depending on God and glorifying Him. Ask God today to make you mindful of Him each time you eat, and seek His guidance concerning quality and quantity.

Lord, forgive me for hoarding food and being greedy. Teach me about eating the foods I should and shouldn't eat. Teach me not to yield to those foods that harm me and cause me to bring dishonor instead of glory to you. Lord, today I am going to give up that second serving to you because I love you. I believe you will bless me for this because you love me.

Total Involvement

And he [Moses] was there with the Lord forty days and forty nights; he did neither eat bread, nor drink water. And he wrote upon the tables the words of the covenant, the ten commandments. (Exod. 34:28)

It is written that God's ways are not our ways, and our ways not His, and how true it is. We see here God sealing His covenant with a fast (a forty-day one, at that) and not a feast as was man's custom of the day. Moses knew God and walked with Him enough to fast and abstain from drink for forty days, depending completely on God to sustain him.

"But that was Moses. He knew God and actually talked with Him audibly. I'm just me!" you say. Well, if you are born again, you have Jesus living in you through His Holy Spirit dwelling in you. You know Him just as well as Moses did because you were bought by Jesus and are a child of the King.

What does all this have to do with dieting or controlled eating? A lot! Moses was so transfixed before God and so involved with Him, that I'm sure he would have considered it blasphemy to say, "Excuse me Lord, I need to have lunch. I'll be back in an hour." In fact, I doubt Moses thought much about food because he was in the presence of Jehovah-God.

When was the last time you were so involved with God that you didn't even think about food? If the answer is never, then you're missing out on some great blessings. Give God a try. Set aside a day to fast, just for Him; not for your diet or to lose an extra couple of pounds, just to worship and commune with God. If you do this with an open heart, in the true spirit of love and giving, your blessings will be far more than just losing one or two pounds. Fasting should be a vital part of our Christian walk. It can be the source of real strength and victory.

Father, just as Moses hungered so for you that he fasted forty days and nights with neither food nor water, show me how to desire you in that way. Teach me what it really means to put you first in my life.

Too Heavy a Burden?

Whence should I have flesh to give unto all this people? for they weep unto me, saying, Give us flesh, that we may eat. (Num. 11:13)

Here is Moses, a man of God, who has walked and talked with the Lord and knows the might and power of Jehovah-God, and he is whimpering to the Lord in self-pity. Does that sound familiar to you? All the people are demanding meat and where can he possibly find that much meat? Then, he compounds his mistake by telling God that he cannot carry everyone because the burden is too heavy for him. He laments, "If this is the way you want to deal with me, let me die."

How like Moses are we? "Not me!" you say. Think about it. How many times have you said to God, "Lord, I can't go on with this diet. Where can I find the strength? It's just too much!" (Some have even wished they were dead.) Well, of course we can't do it. All the self-determination in the world won't get you where you want to go. Only God can be the strength and refuge you need. He desires for you to depend on Him to carry the burden because He knows you don't know how. You make your mistake in trying to do it yourself. All that this accomplishes is frustration and possible anger toward God. Lean on Him; trust Him to carry the burden.

God knew Moses was in a jam and couldn't get out. He also knew that the people were wrong in their requests, and so He didn't become angry with Moses; He understood. Isn't it wonderful that our heavenly Father really does understand even when we wrongfully complain to Him? Search your heart today and ask God's forgiveness for your railings against Him. Admit your own frailty and acknowledge His strength; then live every day in that knowledge, and victory is yours.

Father, forgive me for blaming you so many times for my own lack of faith. I've tried to work things out myself, and when I've failed, I've blamed you. Teach me, Lord, to stand back and see your salvation. All strength and power are yours, Lord, and I lift all my burdens to you and ask you to work the miracles I need.

Looking Back

And say thou unto the people, sanctify yourselves against to morrow and ye shall eat flesh: for ye have wept in the ears of the Lord saying, Who shall give us flesh to eat? for it was well with us in Egypt: therefore the Lord will give you flesh and ye shall eat. Ye shall not eat one day, nor two days, nor five days, neither ten days, nor twenty days; but even a whole month, until it come out of your nostrils, and it be loathsome unto you: because that ye have despised the Lord which is among you, and have wept before him, saying, Why came we forth out of Egypt? (Num. 11:18-20)

The Lord will never force us to do what is good for us and often allows us to go in the path of our own choosing, so we can learn how wrong we are. Here God had been feeding His people from heaven out of His love and desire to care for them. No one was going hungry, but the lusts of the appetite came into play, and the Israelites blew it again. Now, they wanted meat to eat and even wished they had never left Egypt because of the food there. Food became more important to them than God, their freedom, or anything.

Have you been feeling this way? Are you tired of your diet and the restrictions on the food you can eat? Do you long for your "Egypt" (the captivity of complusive eating) because you never had to worry about how much you ate and could fulfill any desire you had? If the answer is yes, don't hate yourself; it is only a temptation just like any other. If you do not entertain the thought, it will vanish. God has given you a diet because it is good for you. And God is so good, He gives lovely fringe benefits like weight loss, better health, healthier skin, more energy, etc. You can't lose with God. Don't go back into bondage for a ham sandwich or a hot fudge sundae. Whether you like it or not, you have a clear choice to make. When you choose, everyone around you will know whom you love most. Be a witness for God and He'll bless you more than eating a hot fudge sundae ever could.

But what if I don't choose God? Well, most likely you'll get what you asked for and then some, and won't like it or yourself very much afterwards. God gave His people quails to eat and they gathered them for several days and stored them for eating. And there was a plague in the camp because of their sin, and many died. The place these people were buried was called Kibroth-hattaavah, or the graves of desire, because their lust (appetite) caused them to sin. Of course, the Lord's prophecy was fulfilled and they ate quail until they were literally sick of it (for God held back the manna).

With us it is no different. If we finally break our word to God and head for the refrigerator, we don't just eat one sandwich like we told God we would. We eat two sandwiches with everything on them, with potato salad or cookies on the side, and then drink a diet soda just to feel justified. How foolish it is to try to fool God.

But that's only the beginning. We really get going with it and head out for an afternoon snack (all afternoon)—a bag of candy here, ice cream there, cake and coffee (black of course, we're watching our weight) at a friend's house (some friend), then comes dinner, and so on. By the time bedtime rolls around, we're either vomiting or wishing we could and we feel sick to our

13

souls because we know we've failed our God, family and friends, and ourselves. That's when we realize that our "Egypt" is not all we remembered it to be. It was sin, shame, and slavery.

God, when I'm tempted by the old life of gluttony and I start asking you to make some small concessions, please say no and remind me of the quails and the Israelites. Remind me what a life of gluttony is really like. Remind me of all the nights I was sick to my stomach or just too stuffed to move, let alone enjoy family and friends. Forgive me for ever considering going back into the bondage of gluttony. Thank you, Lord, for leading me out of "Egypt" and setting me free.

Stoned for Gluttony

And they shall say unto the elders of his city, This our son is stubborn and rebellious, he will not obey our voice; he is a glutton and a drunkard. And all the men of his city shall stone him with stones, that he die: so shalt thou put evil away from among you; and all Israel shall hear, and fear. (Deut. 21:20-21)

If you've ever doubted that gluttony is one of the major sins, this Scripture should shed some new light on the subject. Apparently, God ranked gluttony with rebellion, stubbornness, and drunkenness. You don't think that's so serious? Well, God certainly did, as the punishment was death by stoning. Thank God that we do not have the same rules or three-fourths of America would be stoned to death. How many times have you overindulged with no thought of anyone noticing because everyone else was doing the same thing? Would you have been so openly overindulgent if you had stood out or received harsh disapproval from those around you? No one is punished by others for gluttony (with the exception of a child by a parent and

14

that is not too severe).

Society throughout the world accepts overeating and compulsive eating as a normal way of life, so is it really a sin? Yes, it is a sin because the Lord has ordained it so. He did not create our bodies to function properly under gluttonous conditions, and He knows that physical as well as spiritual discipline is essential to a mature child of God. If you cannot control your appetite, chances are you can easily lose control of other areas of your life. Think of the effect that gluttony and compulsive eating has had on your life. How physically and spiritually healthy are you? How free have you been? How active? If you've answered truthfully, you know that gluttony and compulsive eating is bad news. If you've given it up, thank God and keep the faith. If you haven't, do it now and trust in God to show you that He has a better way. You'll be healthier and happier for it.

Gracious Father, I know gluttony and compulsive eating are wrong. I give it up to you and ask for your perfect control in my appetite. Thank you that we are not subject to the punishment of the Old Testament, but are under the grace of the blood of Jesus Christ. Forgive me for taking gluttony so lightly when you deem it so serious. I ask this in Jesus' name and I thank you for the protection, strength, and victory in Him.

Take Nothing Home

When thou comest into thy neighbour's vineyard, then thou mayest eat grapes thy fill at thine own pleasure; but thou shall not put any in thy vessel. (Deut. 23:24)

This was one of the numerous civil laws given the children of Israel and it expresses such deep wisdom on God's part. He

15

wanted His people to be loving and compassionate to one another, so He allowed a person to eat from another's vineyard if he were passing by and hungry. This part of the law teaches giving and providing for the needs of others. Then, God put a stipulation or two on the rule. First, they could only eat their fill, not any more, and second, they could not take any home with them. The first part, of course, discourages gluttony, and the second both discourages gluttony and saw to it that no one stole part of another's crop to sell for his own gain.

Of course, the gluttony aspect is directly related to our situation. How often we've been a guest for dinner, a party, or a gathering, and enjoyed some food or dessert so much we wanted to take some home with us even though we were stuffed at the moment. We'd tell ourselves it would be for tomorrow or even for some other member of the family (in which case we take two servings, so one is still left for us). The hostess is usually gracious enough to give it to us, but at times we snitch some without even asking (especially if it's a large banquet). Generally the food never makes it to the next day. The glutton gets home and shoves it down (unless of course he has over-stuffed to the point of not being able to get another bite in, but for the true glutton, this is a rare occasion).

We can benefit from this law God gave His people by using it as a rule-of-thumb when we go to a neighbor's or some social occasion where food is served. Let's eat (permitted food only, of course) to our fill, not to overflowing; then let's call it quits. If it was good and you enjoyed it, compliment the person responsible, but remember that tomorrow is another day with other food. Don't take any leftovers home. Why? Because you are subjecting yourself to unnecessary temptation, and with the taste of that food still clear in your mind, you may yield to the temptation and spoil the great victory you just experienced at the dinner or banquet.

When such a special occasion is scheduled, talk to God ahead of time. Promise Him before you go, before you see all those tempting goodies, that you won't take anything home. Then keep your word to God no matter how great the temptation. Believe me, when you get home again, you'll be shouting for joy and praising God because of the victory you've experienced, so remember to thank Him for it!

Lord, when I'm in a situation that calls for eating at someone else's home, help me to go to you first. I make a commitment to you to eat only my allowed foods unless none of them are present, then I'll eat the least harmful in small amounts. Father, remind me when I've eaten my fill and don't let me overeat. When it is time to leave, I'll not bring food home with me because that is a gluttonous act for me, and I am healed of gluttony in Jesus' name.

Not Your Strength

And the Lord, he it is that doth go before thee; he will be with thee, he will not fail thee, neither forsake thee: fear not, neither be dismayed. (Deut. 31:8)

These were the words of comfort and truth Moses gave the Israelites shortly before they crossed into the promised land. He knew he would not be there to strengthen and encourage them, so he tried to assure them ahead of time. God is always with us and at the same time He goes before us to fight our battles. God doesn't lose nor does He leave us stranded. God brought the people of Israel through the desert forty years (a lot longer than they planned, but they were slow learners) and He never forsook them even when they turned on Him.

It is no different with us. If you've been in the diet desert a lot longer than you would like to, maybe it's because you have not been ready to step over into the promised land of God's normal weight and eating for you. Perhaps you've been a bit rebellious and have not learned to trust Him enough. Don't give up. We have God's assurance that He is with us and will prepare a way out for us. God knows before you sit down at the table what kind of battle will be waged and He is faithful to offer you a battle plan if you only ask. No enemy is too great, no temptation too strong, that God can't handle it for you.

Suppose you are down to your correct weight and are on the threshold of entering the promised land, but are afraid once you get there you'll blow it. What should you do? The same thing you did while you were in the desert places. Lean on the Lord because only He can give you power over temptation. Don't depend on your own self-discipline and will power to win. If you do, you'll lose sooner or later (most likely sooner). Purpose in your heart to call on Him before you give in and you'll not fail.

Father, teach me all I need to know while I'm in the desert. Don't let me out one second early because I don't want to go back again. I know fear is not from you, and I will not be afraid of any temptations or tests because I know you are both with me and have gone before me to prepare my victorious battle plan. Thank you, Lord, that you are with me in the desert and in the promised land, so that I can enjoy my freedom from gluttony and the blessings of a new life.

Too Much of a Good Thing

He made him ride on the high places of the earth, that he might eat the increase of the fields; and he made him to suck honey out of the rock, and oil out of the flinty rock; Butter of kine, and milk of sheep, with fat of lambs, and rams of the breed of Bashan, and goats, with the fat of kidneys of wheat, and thou didst drink the pure blood of the grape. But Jeshurun waxed fat, and kicked: thou art waxen fat, thou art grown thick, thou art covered with fatness; then he forsook God which made him, and lightly esteemed the Rock of his salvation. (Deut. 32:13-15)

Israel was given the "good life" by God, the same life He wants to give us today. All the foods listed above are good foods—good for health and strength and growth. If they were not good, God would not have given them so freely. Then why did Israel grow fat? Because even good food is bad when it is eaten to excess. This is the underlying fallacy of health food. No food is healthy in excess, except spiritual food (which apparently the Israelites did not overindulge in). God gave them all of this and they went overboard with their appetites again. They did not call on God or recall what they were taught in the desert, but went right ahead growing fat in their gluttony and their excess of worldly appetite.

"Jeshurun" is a term of endearment for Israel. Isn't God loving? Even though they had sinned, turned from Him, and He was angry with them, He still loved them. He's that way with us, too. Have you ever made it to your promised land, overeaten and grown fat again, putting God on the side and forgetting His salvation? Most dieters have been in this place many times, especially if they have not discovered God's perfect way to be free from gluttony and compulsive eating. Does God forsake you? No, He may allow you some rough times until your rebellion is eliminated, but He still won't leave you.

Whether you're on a diet or a maintenance eating plan, it is important to remember that good foods are only good in the correct amounts. Let God control your eating the rest of your time on earth. Don't wax fat and forget Him. He loves you.

Heavenly Father, show me the amount of food I need. Teach me to enjoy but not overenjoy those good things you've provided. Lord, forgive me if I've begun to forget you and to go my own way. Keep me on the right eating plan and ever mindful that you are my total salvation in Jesus.

Weaned from Manna

> And they did eat of the old corn of the land on the morrow after the passover, unleavened cakes, and parched corn in the selfsame day. And the manna ceased on the morrow after they had eaten of the old corn of the land; neither had the children of Israel manna any more; but they did eat of the fruit of the land of Canaan that year. (Josh. 5:11-12)

God has a purpose in everything He does and His ways are so wonderfully marvelous. When we wean a baby from milk to solid food, it is because he is strong enough to take the solid food. In fact, if solid food (a change of diet) is not given, the child will not grow stronger. He will be sickly and perhaps even die.

When the Israelites reached the promised land, their diet was changed, too, because they needed to grow more. God did not want to milk-feed them with manna forever. He wanted them to go on to better things. So, He gave them the food of the land of Canaan to eat. Of course we've seen that they eventually misused this food, but still they grew and learned.

While we're dieting, God has our food greatly restricted in amount and content. He knows that now we are mature enough to know what is good for us, and so He gives us a food plan to meet our needs and to teach us things we must know to really grow in Him when we reach the promised land.

Learn all you can while in the desert; that's why you are there. When you reach the promised land, you'll be strong enough and mature enough for a change of diet. God will more than likely allow a greater variety of food and perhaps a larger amount. Be in tune to His will concerning these things. This could be the beginning of a new life for you if you grow strong in Him as your body grows trim and healthy in His plan of eating for you.

If you find it wearisome to eat God's "manna" day after day, remember that when you learn to be content with God's food, He will increase the variety, and place it in its rightful place of priority in your life—if you will let Him.

Father, how exciting it is to know that you are bottle-feeding me so I can grow stronger and firmer and healthier. Thank you for the "manna" because I know it is good for me and will sustain me, while I am learning that food should be pleasant and satisfying but not tempting. Lord, show me how to make the transition from "milk" to "meat" both physically and spiritually.

Sacrifice for Another

And Boaz said unto her, At mealtime come thou hither, and eat of the bread, and dip thy morsel in the vinegar. And she sat beside the reapers and he reached her parched corn, and she did eat, and was sufficed, and left. . . . So she gleaned in the field until even, and beat out that she had gleaned: and it was about an ephah of barley. And she took it up and went into the city: and her mother in law saw what she had gleaned: and she brought forth, and gave to her that she had reserved after she was sufficed. (Ruth 2:14, 17-18)

How long have you been a glutton? If you've been healed of it, how long were you a glutton? Remember your attitude toward food? Although you stuffed it into your mouth freely, when it came to sharing, that was another matter. You weren't so free with it. How many times did you hoard that last serving of your favorite food or greedily hope at dinner no one else would want seconds of a certain food even before you had finished the portion on your plate? Only you can give truthful answers to these questions and, if you're guilty and haven't repented or if you're possessive of your "diet" food, you need to confess your sin and seek forgiveness in Jesus' name.

So many of us were gluttons for so long we aren't able to discern proper behavior for a temperate person. Ruth is a classic biblical example of a temperate, God-loving person. Most of us would have thought Ruth crazy (and maybe some of us did) back in our gluttonous days. She went into the field at sunrise and would have worked all day without food and without a word.

Now this would have been enough for most of us to have guessed that the sun had gotten to her head, but she just continued doing silly things. She is offered lunch by Boaz, but she only eats what she needs and saves the rest, and then works until evening. She doesn't eat what she saved, but she just beats out her barley and heads home to Naomi with an ephah of barley and her "munchies." Now, we figure we've guessed it. She takes a nice hot bath, lets Naomi have the barley, and then she'll enjoy her food while she's relaxing. Aren't we surprised when she hands Naomi the barley and the remainder of her lunch. What was it about Ruth that made her do such a strange thing? Sure, we outwardly admire her, but inside we didn't really think she was too smart.

The key to Ruth is love and self-sacrifice. She was obviously a temperate person and in control of her appetite, but it took more than that to resist eating to her fill in that position. Even the most temperate person in the world would have been tempted to eat all the lunch. I'm sure Ruth *was* tempted, but the important thing is that she resisted that temptation. She knew in her heart that her love for Naomi was more important than one day of hunger. She knew there would be other days and she would have food, but she knew this day it was important for her to sacrifice for another.

How does that apply to us? Very directly! As a glutton we eat as if there is no tomorrow (and sometimes no next meal). Even when we know we are hurting our temple of the Holy Spirit, we don't care enough to sacrifice. We hurt our families, our health, and our own hearts, but still we are not willing to sacrifice.

If you've been healed of gluttony or compulsive eating, but keep backsliding, think of Ruth and then think of someone you could sacrifice for (God would be the best choice). Do it as a love offering to Him. Actually give up a meal. Then, begin to eat each meal with the attitude of: "What do I really *need* to eat and what could I leave for someone else or until tomorrow?" Ask the Lord for His help over the temptation to overeat. He will not turn you away.

Father, I've always resented the Ruths of this world because they seem to be able to give up food so easily, and I can't even when I want to. Heal me, Lord, and deliver me from gluttony [if He has, thank Him here] in Jesus' name. Thank you for forgiving me. I want to go on now with you to become like Ruth, not just outside but inside. Lord, I want it to come from the heart, and I know you will help me in this battle.

Good Psychology, Bad Bible

And when all the people came to cause David to eat meat while it was yet day, David sware, saying, So do God to me, and more also, if I taste bread, or ought else, till the sun be down. (2 Sam. 3:35)

David was fasting and mourning the death of Abner, who had come to David in peace and was sent away in peace but was killed by one of David's men to avenge his brother, whom

Abner had killed. David mourned because he had sent him away in peace and safety as a friend, and he was murdered by one of David's men. The Scripture says that David even wept, so you know he was sad and shaken by this.

Now David's people came to him to console him, so what did they offer him—food. It was a typical case of "Eat this; you'll feel much better." We've all experienced this in our lives, and it's so wrong. Even today, after a funeral, what do people do? Bring food over for the family of the deceased. When we were sick, what did our parents do? Give us ice cream or some special food to make us feel better. The one you love drops you, so what does your best friend suggest? "Let's make some cookies." And on and on it goes! It may be good psychology, but it isn't good Bible, nor is it God's will. Any time we turn first to anything besides Him for strength and consolation, we are making that person or thing an idol. Most of us readily accept the pleasurable fleshly substitute for God's perfect peace and consolation, but David did not.

David was a man of God who knew the value of putting his physical comfort aside in order to receive total comfort from God. He refused the meat until the appointed time of sundown; this was his agreement to God and he kept it. I'm sure it would have been easier to drown his sorrows in a big meal, but his soul would have still been starving and he knew it. He stayed and fed his soul first and by sundown he was able to handle the eating properly, for reasons of hunger, not consolation.

Let's learn how to say no to those bribes all our well-meaning friends and relatives try to push on us. When you've had a bad day at work and your spouse says, "Let's go out to dinner and you can have whatever you want to eat; you can diet tomorrow," learn to say, "No, that won't change my bad day, only Jesus can." Take your leave and go to that prayer closet of yours and contact God first. Let Him minister to you as only He can because He knows your needs. Then if your spouse still wants to take you to dinner, you can go and enjoy acceptable food and not even break your diet. It may sound the least enjoyable of the two choices, but believe me, it's the best. When you choose God, it's always the best.

Lord, when you see me running to food to solve bad feelings, problems, worries, stop me and remind me that food (good or bad food) can only complicate the situation by adding guilt and self-condemnation. Father, I know you are the answer to everything. You can solve any situation that is bothering me; food can only cover it up or compound it. Help me to learn to always choose you.

No Contradictions

For so was it charged me by the word of the Lord, saying, Eat no bread, nor drink water, nor turn again by the same way that thou camest. . . . Then he [the prophet] said unto him, Come home with me, and eat bread. And he said, I may not return with thee, nor go in with thee; neither will I eat bread nor drink water with thee in this place: For it was said to me by the word of the Lord, Thou shalt eat no bread nor drink water there, nor turn again to go by the way that thou camest. He said unto him, I am a prophet also as thou art; and an angel spake unto me by the word of the Lord saying Bring him back with thee unto thine house, that he may eat bread and drink water. But he lied unto him. So he went back with him, and did eat bread in his house, and drank water. (1 Kings 13:9, 15-19)

Here was a man of God who was given a direct order not to eat, drink, or deviate from the way God told him to go. He heard from God and had his orders, so when the prophet tempted him with food, drink, and lodging, he said "no thank you" and told him what God had said. But apparently his whole heart wasn't in it because with a few simple words from the prophet, he relented. Now you say, "Well, the prophet lied and told the man of God he had heard from the Lord, so it wasn't really the man's fault." Wrong! He was a man of God, also a prophet, and he knew that God did not go back on His word nor contradict himself. Nevertheless he believed a lie and as soon as he had eaten and drunk, the Lord prophesied through the prophet that the man of God would die and not be buried in the tomb of his ancestors, and it came to pass.

How many times has God established eating rules for us, and we go along resisting the temptations put before us until one day in our heart we wish someone would say, "God told me to tell you it's all right to break that diet today." That's all the convincing we need. We forget that God doesn't work that way. He gave the order directly to you for a reason, and He won't go back on His word, especially through someone else. But when you've transgressed and eaten, then you know (just like Adam and Eve) that you blew it. Thank God His punishment isn't sudden death, but we do gain weight. Ask His forgiveness and go on remembering next time not to be so easily led astray.

Lord, search my heart and expose all those wrong desires I have. Don't let me fall into a trap because of sinful motivation. I know you are true to your word; teach me to be also.

Give to Receive

And she said, As the Lord thy God liveth, I have not cake, but an hand full of meal in a barrel, and a little oil in a cruse: and behold I am gathering two sticks, that I may go in and dress it for me and my son, that we may eat it, and die. And Elijah said unto her, Fear not, go and do as thou hast said: but make me thereof a little cake first, and bring it unto me, and after make for thee and for thy son. For thus saith the Lord God of Israel, The barrel of meal shall not waste, neither shall the cruse of oil fail, until the day that the Lord sendeth rain upon the earth. And she went and did according to the saying of Elijah: and she, and her house, did eat many days. (1 Kings 17:12-15)

There was a drought in the land, and this widow and her son had obviously come to the end of their food reserve and were going to eat their last meal and wait for death. Then, Elijah came along and asked the woman to share with him all that they had left and to serve him first, and if she did, that the Lord would provide. The woman did so, and she, her family, and Elijah ate many days and the oil and the meal did not run out, just as God had promised.

This is a story of faith and giving, not just giving food, but giving of one's self. What would you do if a stranger asked for the last food that you had in the house when you knew that you had no way of getting more? Would you give to him or would you esteem yourself more important? It is this kind of sacrificial giving that God desires His children to have. So many times we are reminded in the Scripture that we must give if we desire to receive. God works that way with regulating our eating also. If we'll give to Him the foods that He tells us we shouldn't have or just wants us to give Him as a sacrifice, then He will not only give us the weight loss results (if we're in need of them) but will give us the right food in the right quantity and will see to it that it satisfies us. He will give us life through His food instead of the early death we were going to have with ours.

Father, teach me to give of myself to you and to others as well as give up foods, beverages, habits, etc., that are harmful to me or others. Lord, I'm going to give and I'm depending on you to help me receive the good things you have for me—like healthy food and self-control. I ask and pray this in Jesus' name.

Quantity is Not Quality

> And the angel of the Lord came again the second time, and touched him and said, Arise and eat; because the journey is too great for thee. And he arose, and did eat and drink, and went in the strength of that meat forty days and forty nights unto Horeb the mount of God. (1 Kings 19:7-8)

Elijah was fleeing Jezebel and Ahab who sought his life, and was asleep in the wilderness when an angel awoke him and gave him bread and water to eat and he fell asleep again. This occurred again, only this time he ate and journeyed forty days and forty nights on that food.

How often have you told yourself that your diet is too low in calories or amount, or your eating plan is too restrictive. In fact, haven't we all said, "A person can't live this way! It's unhealthy!" Isn't it amusing that the only time a dieter worries about nutrition is when he can use it as an excuse to go back to overindulging. We always forget nutrition when we are gorging ourselves (probably because we assume with all we eat we must surely get all the nutrition we need). This is a lie we tell ourselves because we don't want to face the fact that most of what we eat is low in nutrition, high in calories and carbohydrates, and is so full of junk and additives that it is harmful to our bodies. The irony is that the restricted eating or smaller quantity diet usually creates a situation in which we need less food to carry us from meal to meal and, because we eat less, we have more energy and are more active. The person who says that such eating is too hard or unhealthy can't even make it from one huge meal to the other without stuffing down a snack (junk food usually) and they barely have the get-up-and-go to fix their own food. Also, their physical ailments are usually greater and more pronounced.

Don't try to fool yourself; face the truth that is in your heart. You know God's way is best and He would never give you any eating plan that was harmful to you. After all, He's your Creator and knows the best foods and habits to get and keep your body functioning at its best level.

You really don't need as much bulk food as you think you do. Elijah went forty days and nights on what he ate and Christian men and women today still do the same when called by God. If this can be done, how much more can we live from day to day on less bulk and more nutritious food?

Father, I've lied to myself and you all these years. I know that quality has nothing to do with quantity. I know I've polluted my body for many years with junk foods, and even the good foods I've eaten, I've overindulged in. Forgive me, Lord, in Jesus' name. Now, show me the amount of food I need to be healthy, not how much I can have and still not be a glutton. I know I have to stop thinking greedily and start thinking and acting in moderation. Thank you for ministering to me today.

Death in the Pot

So they poured out for the men to eat. And it came to pass, as they were eating of the pottage, that they cried out and said, O thou man of God, there is death in the pot. And they could not eat thereof. (2 Kings 4:40)

Some of Elisha's servants had gathered herbs to make pottage for Elisha and the people with him, but apparently someone had gathered poisonous herbs and someone perceived it in time and cried out a warning, ". . . there's death in the pot." How often has God called out to us that there was death in the pot, on the plate, in the refrigerator, at the bakery, the fast-food restaurant, etc? How many times have we listened to Him or even heard Him? Even when a doctor tells a glutton that he's eating himself to death, he doesn't listen.

God is sending out a loud cry to His people today, warning them, "There's death in the pot." We are putting garbage by the pound into our bodies each day that was never meant to be there and is harmful. God wants us to turn away from those harmful foods and back to His good food from the earth that He has provided. He also wants us to regulate the quantity of food as well as the quality. Too much of a good thing is still bad. Next time you eat something, wait upon the Lord and ask, "Lord, is there death in the pot? Is this good for me or harmful?"

Lord, forgive me for all the times I've failed to hear your warnings about the foods I was eating. Even when they made me violently ill, I wouldn't turn them loose. Only you can set me free. Teach me to grow closer to you and to heed your warnings about food and anything else that isn't good for me.

Lean on the Lord

Ye shall not need to fight in this battle: set yourselves, stand ye still, and see the salvation of the Lord with you, O Judah and Jerusalem: fear not, nor be dismayed; to morrow go out against them: for the Lord will be with you. (2 Chron. 20:17)

Have you been fighting the "battle of the bulge" and losing it? Do you keep asking for God's help and still fail? Perhaps you've been trying to work it out yourself, and that's why you haven't won. Have you been looking to your diet for weight loss? Have you been looking to your own self-discipline for self-control in eating? Have you been looking to certain foods as good for health and still feeling poorly? If the answer is yes to any or all of these questions, then you're trying to win the battle yourself.

You must realize it is more of a spiritual battle than a physical one. Of course, the outward problem is physical, and certain physical measures must be taken to remedy this. However, the true problem is lack of control and discipline of the appetite because of attempts to do things without God being in control. Satan is there to see to it that you remain in the same "diet trap" just like a yo-yo—you lose, then gain, then lose. Just when you think you have it made, a small, gluttonous thought enters your mind and you break because it's just between you and the tempter; you aren't allowing God to fight. Of course, we have to do our part, but how wonderful to know that when we're losing and can't go on, we can stop, stand still, and see the salvation of God as He wins a battle we know our flesh never could.

If you're a loser today, call on God; then when the tempter comes, stand back, yield the situation to God, and rejoice in the victory.

Father, I realize now that I've been trying to do it all myself, and that's why I've continued to fail. Lord, I confess I can't do it, and I call on you to win the battle for me. I'm standing back Lord; show me your excellent salvation!

Feast Days

Then he said unto them, Go your way, eat the fat, and drink the sweet, and send portions unto them for whom nothing is prepared: for this day is holy unto our Lord: neither be ye sorry; for the joy of the Lord is your strength. (Neh. 8:10)

Ezra had just read the law of God to the people from the book of Moses and the people wept as they understood the words, but Nehemiah told them not to weep, but rejoice for it was a holy day to them, and a day of celebration. He instructed them to go out and eat "rich food and sweet drinks" (New English Bible). Is this contrary to God's will? Of course not! There are feast days when rich and sweet food is acceptable, but still only in proper quantity. Don't think that just because you are on a diet or have had a problem with compulsive eating, that you can never enjoy food again because it is sinful. When you are walking in victory and can control your urge to succumb to gluttonous temptation, then you too can enjoy feast days and special occasions, but with a different concept.

Some foods will never be good for you and perhaps God will take them away permanently, but for the most part, you'll be able to enjoy the holidays in moderation. God understands and approves of rejoicing on feast days. He doesn't want you mourning when everyone else is glad, but wants you to enjoy in moderation those special times for special foods.

Father, how wonderful it is to know you understand and want us to enjoy the feast days too. But it is more sweet to know that your joy is my strength, not food. Thank you, Lord, that I can feast on your love and your Word every day and grow strong and healthy in you.

Remember the Giver

So the children went in and possessed the land, and thou subduedst before them the inhabitants of the land, the Canaanites, and gavest them into their hands, with their kings, and the people of the land, that they might do with them as they would. And they took strong cities, and a fat land, and possessed houses full of all goods, wells digged, vineyards, and oliveyards, and fruit trees in abundance: so they did eat, and were filled, and became fat, and delighted themselves in thy great goodness. Nevertheless they were disobedient, and rebelled against thee, and cast thy law behind their backs, and slew thy prophets which testified against them to turn them to thee, and they wrought great provocations. (Neh. 9:24-26)

God is always winning battles for His people because He wants them to be free and have an abundant life here on earth. He wants the best for His own, but He asks in return that they love, obey, and worship Him. He won this great victory for His people and gave them Canaan and all the good things that they didn't even have to work for, and they took these and enjoyed the bounty of them until they grew fat and loved the possessions God had given them more than God.

People don't seem to change much basically through the ages. God blesses us with health, wealth, food, two cars, etc., and we forget the source and worship the gifts. The glutton is especially guilty of this because he truly doesn't care to listen to God's rules concerning his sin. God provides the food for him, and he abuses it by overindulging day after day. This is not God's will. Sure, He wants you to have enough to eat and good food to eat, but He doesn't want the desire and the love for these things to exceed our love and desire for Him and His laws. Examine your life and see if you've possessed any "land" God has given you and then made it your god.

Father, thank you for the good things of this earth which you've provided. I know you want the best for me, but, Father, I want you. Give me more love and desire for you first, then give me these other things, that I might delight in your laws and worship you.

Fasting is Important

Go, gather together all the Jews that are present in Shushan, and fast ye for me, and neither eat nor drink three days, night or day: I also and my maidens will fast likewise; and so will I go in unto the king, which is not according to the law: and if I perish, I perish. (Esther 4:16)

Esther was fighting for her life and the life of every Jew in the country, as a decree had come forth that all Jews be killed on a certain day. She knew the situation was critical and drastic measures were needed, so she called on the power of fasting and prayer to God. She could have just spent a few hours or even a day in prayer and then gone to the king, but apparently she didn't feel that was sufficient for the gravity of this situation. So, she called for three days of fasting and prayer, and then said, "I'll go in and if I perish, I'll perish." She knew she had done all she could.

Do you have a problem today that's important to you? Perhaps you're fat and need to lose weight. Perhaps you keep failing at your diet. Perhaps you can't seem to stop eating those foods God has convicted you about. Maybe you're a glutton and just don't have the strength to stop, but you hate yourself for it. Whatever your problem is today, nothing is too big for God. But He wants you to convince Him you really want to get out of your situation. Why not try prayer and fasting to God? There is dramatic power in the two of them together, and what better approach for someone with an eating problem. Set aside some time, plan ahead and then go before the Lord with all your heart, and you'll be blessed and given the solution and strength you need for victory over your situation. Esther got powerful results. She not only saved herself and her people, but she exposed the true enemy of the king and restored her uncle to favor with the king.

God, thank you for showing me the importance of prayer and fasting. I realize now, no problem is too great for you to solve. Thank you for helping me to grow in you today.

The Trials of Job

Teach me, and I will hold my tongue: and cause me to understand wherein I have erred. (Job 6:24)

In Job's efforts to understand why all these terrible things were happening to him, he never blamed God for his situation. He knew he was a man of God and felt he had done no wrong, yet something had caused this difficulty in his life. Never did he assume it was God's fault, but instead said, "Tell me what I've done wrong, and I'll straighten it out."

Has Satan been giving you a hard time? Have you been "starving" but not losing any weight? Do you have trouble convincing people that you've really given up that old way of eating? Have diverse problems entered your life seemingly because you've followed God in your eating situation? Do you, like Job, wonder if you're on the wrong track or have missed God's way for you? You may not have missed God, but probably are right on target and the devil doesn't like it one bit! Remember, God is right there with you always and He allows trials and temptations to come your way to test and refine your faith in Him. If you truly can't think of any disobedience on your part, then get happy over those problems because it's exam time and you can pass with straight A's. Hold on and trust in God; the end results are well worth it. Just look at the last chapter of Job.

Praise you, Father, for allowing these trials to come my way. I know I grow stronger through them and win the victory over them in Jesus' name. Teach me to be patient and if I have erred, show me that I might confess and repent of it.

Satan Will Attack

> If iniquity be in thine hand, put it far away, and let not wickedness dwell in thy tabernacles. For then shalt thou lift up thy face without spot; yea, thou shall be stedfast, and shalt not fear: Because thou shalt forget thy misery, and remember it as waters that pass away. (Job 11:14-16)

It seems almost like Job had the dieter in mind when he uttered those words. We were walking in iniquity when we were gluttons (fatties, compulsive eaters, etc.), but we put it away (you should if you haven't) and cleansed our tabernacles (our bodies) of the wrong. Now confessing alone isn't cleansing, neither is repentance. In order for our bodies to be completely cleansed, we must confess our sin, repent, and then remove all signs and results of that sin, i.e., fat, bad eating habits, incorrect foods, etc. This is what the diet process is all about, cleansing the body, and of course it is not easy. At times we are so tired of it, we want to quit, but that's just Satan's high-pressure tactics. We must go on and finish the job of cleaning our temples to please God as well as have more liveable bodies.

It seems sometimes as if we'll never reach the end, but we will, and when we do, Job says we'll forget all the bad and hard times and remember it like water under the bridge (and Job should know). Think back on other trials and hard times in your life. Isn't it painless to remember the ones you were victorious over because it all worked out okay in the end? A mother suffers in childbirth, but a year later when her child is walking, she can barely remember what it was like to be pregnant. So it is with our battle. When it's over, even the bad will be remembered as having worth.

Lord, you know it's hard for me now and it seems like the cleansing will never end, but I know it will. Thank you for showing me that when you win the victory, all of this will just be water under the bridge. I can lead a happy, comfortable, healthy life on your food, being satisfied far beyond anything I could imagine with the old way, because you are the one who satisfies. Thank you, Father, in the sweet name of Jesus.

Clean Hands

The righteous also shall hold on his way, and he that hath clean hands shall be stronger and stronger. (Job 17:9)

Did you know that if you are a born-again believer you are righteous? But you say, "I fall so often and sadden God, how can I be righteous?" Well, of yourself you can't, but Jesus through His precious blood has made you righteous where you could not be. Therefore, you are righteous in God's eyes and should keep going in His way. When you are moving with God, don't allow yourself to be moved by anyone else. If God has given you an eating plan, don't abandon it because someone tells you it isn't good for your health or that they know a plan that's better and gets faster results. There is no plan better than God's plan for you personally; it *is* the best.

This Scripture also has another beautiful truth, and that is, if your hands are clean (i.e., you are free from guilt and unconfessed sin) you'll grow stronger. Are your hands clean today in the area of eating or are there traces of chocolate frosting or potato chip oil on them? If you have been sneaking a little bit here and a little bit there (you know, a taste won't hurt), then don't be surprised when you seem to be getting weaker.

Your hands aren't clean—you won't grow stronger. Confess your weakness, clean your hands and stand righteous before God. Then your strength and will power will increase in the area of food and you can charge ahead into victory.

Father, I thank you today for making me righteous through the blood of Jesus; I am so undeserving. Forgive me for not having truly clean hands (as far as food goes), in Jesus' name. I realize now that one taste of forbidden food (remember Adam and Eve) is just as sinful as a whole portion. Lord, my hands are washed and clean now; strengthen me through all of this as I go on in your will.

Preferring God's Word

Neither have I gone back from the commandment of his lips; I have esteemed the words of his mouth more than my necessary food. (Job 23:12)

What a wonderful testimony this is to the dieter and former compulsive eater or glutton. How sweet it is to say that you value God's Word more than necessary food—not just pleasurable but necessary food. This is how we should all value the Word of God, for it is through His Word that we live. Without physical food, the body would grow weak and die, but only the lack of God's Word (spiritual food) will cause atrophy of the spirit and soul.

Today, face this issue in your life. How much do you esteem God's Word to you? Enough to stick to your diet? That's good! Enough to turn down that piece of cake your family has offered? That's better! Enough to abstain from eating because permitted food is not available (even if you haven't eaten all day and everyone else is ordering food to eat at one of your favorite old spots)? That's best! When you reach the point of choosing to give up eating if that's what it takes to keep God's Word to you, then you've really esteemed His Word more than your necessary food.

Lord, how precious your words are to me, but I have not yet esteemed them more than my necessary food. Give me that chance, for I know that I will be blessed greatly when I have this truth deeply in my heart.

You Can Enjoy Food

He openeth also their ear to discipline, and commandeth that they return from iniquity. If they obey and serve him, they shall spend their days in prosperity, and their years in pleasures. (Job 36:10-11)

Since God has convicted you about food and eating habits, have you begun to feel that the pleasure of eating is a sin? Do you feel a little guilty when you really enjoy a meal even when you didn't break your diet or overeat? If the answer is yes, it isn't surprising nor is it unusual, but it is wrong thinking. Often when Satan can't get us to break our agreement to God concerning eating, he tries another approach to make us miserable; it's called "the guilt trip." He tells you you're being sinful and lustful toward food because you really enjoyed that meal, and that you really haven't changed inside. He tells you you're still the same old glutton you always were. He's the father of liars; this is just his underhanded approach to stealing the victory from you.

God has given you an eating plan and a selection of foods that is both good and good for you. He never intended that your meals be without pleasure, only that they be temperate and that your desire be healthy, not lustful. God opened your ears and you heard Him discipline you in this area. You obeyed Him and turned to Him and served Him. Job says that you should expect years of prosperity and pleasure. God wants you to enjoy all of the good things He's provided. He only asks that you not set your heart on them. So enjoy your food, but enjoy the Lord first. Honor His wishes that you might live in honest prosperity and pleasure.

God, you are so gracious to provide for me not only a healthy eating plan, but one I can enjoy properly without sinning against you. I realize now my guilt concerning enjoying the food you provided was just a trick to get me to condemn myself and eventually to quit altogether on my diet. Lord, thank you for revealing this to me and renewing my strength.

Concentrate on God's Word

Blessed is the man that walketh not in the counsel of the ungodly, nor standeth in the way of sinners, nor sitteth in the seat of the scornful. But his delight is in the law of the Lord; And in his law does he meditate day and night. And he shall be like a tree planted by the rivers of water, that bringeth forth his fruit in his season; his leaf also shall not wither: and whatsoever he doeth shall prosper. (Ps. 1:1-3)

How wonderful is this promise of God and how beneficial to us if we can seize it and appropriate it for ourselves.

First we are told we are blessed if we don't act on the advice of an ungodly person or operate as sinners do. What does this mean to the dieter? This means not to take the advice of someone you know is ungodly. This does not only mean personal friends, but doctors, or even books written by ungodly men. It may seem to get you results, but most of it won't last and much of the philosophy behind those diets is against God's Word concerning temperance. Many diets encourage you to overeat certain foods to help you lose weight. If it transgresses the Word of God, it is ungodly. If you must get human advice, go to a Christian who you know is a godly person and still compare his advice to God's Word to see if it lines up.

The promise says to meditate on God's Word day and night. Dieter, I can think of no better way to resist temptation and continue growing stronger than to meditate on God's Word, for it is through meditation on the Word that it becomes real to you and you transfer it from your head to your heart. When you have a battle to fight or you're on your way to dinner and you know the temptation will be great, spend some time in God's Word preparing for the battle. There is no more powerful weapon than the Word of God.

If you do, the Word says you'll be like a well-watered tree. You'll have a healthy body and spirit, and people will know it by the fruit you produce. Your body will slim down and that will prove to others you have been keeping God's Word You'll be stronger spiritually in all areas and temptations will be fewer because of your strength in Jesus. Also, whatever you do (within God's will, of course) will prosper. That's quite a reward just for doing what we should do for God, wouldn't you say? Start claiming that promise in your life today and see the results.

God, thank you for this wonderful promise. I claim it in my life and will not walk in the counsel of the ungodly. I will meditate on your Word and will place it in my heart that I might walk in your way. I want to be like a well-watered tree and produce your good fruit and prosper. Thank you, Lord, for the results; I know you are faithful to fulfill your Word.

Least Painful Way

The Lord is the portion of mine inheritance and of my
cup: thou maintainest my lot. (Ps. 16:5)

Does it sometimes seem like the heathen are prospering and
doing so well and you are doing so poorly, even though you are
following God? Looks can be deceiving! The Word says that
God is looking after you and keeping your life. He is your
inheritance and that means all good things belong to you,
especially a trim, healthy body. When you see heathens doing
better on their "quicky" diets than you are on yours, remember,
God is taking you through this diet slowly because it is easier on
your body. He is teaching and correcting the real problems you
have that have resulted in fatness and gluttony. When He is
finished with you, it will be over, and you will be completely
healed once and for all if you continue in His will. Most of the
heathen will live on the diet yo-yo the rest of their lives, gaining
and losing and enduring forever the physical and mental
anguish (that you once knew so well). So when you're scoffed
at, just smile and say, "Thank you, Jesus, that you're taking me
through this in the least painless way."

Father, how wonderful it is that you've provided for every
area of my life. I realize that if I learn my lessons the first time as
you teach me concerning food and eating habits, I'll never have
to deal with the self-condemnation, humiliation, and anguish
again. Thank you, Father, in Jesus' name for this help and
assurance.

Make No Demands

The meek shall eat and be satisfied: They shall praise
the Lord that seek him: Your heart shall live forever.
(Ps. 22:26)

When you entered your diet or eating plan, did you enter in meekness or did you have a whole list of things that God had to allow or provide? Have you been satisfied with your eating plan? If you haven't, perhaps it's because you didn't enter in meekness. David said the meek shall eat and be satisfied. Are you seeking God? Do you praise Him?

Gluttony and wrong eating have plagued this country for so many years that it is an accepted way of life by many. Have you ever been poor, really poor? When you're poor, you sit down and eat whatever food is provided, and you're more than thankful for that. You don't push away a plate of beans and rice when your stomach is empty and say, "No thanks, I don't want it. I'd like some filet mignon." You eat and are satisfied to be full. You know that what is there is the best that could be provided. We can all learn from this attitude because it is how we should feel toward the food God has provided—both thankful and sure that it is His best for us in this situation. Of course, God is not poor and could give us steak everyday, but He must provide only what is good for us. Even good food is not always good for us. When we can accept the fact that God has provided the quality and quantity of food for us that is good for our particular need, then we can eat in meekness and be satisfied. We can truly seek Him in a spirit of praise and thanksgiving and have everlasting hearts with which to love Him.

Father, you are the great Jehovah-Jirah (God provides) and have met my needs with this eating plan. Forgive me, in Jesus' name, for complaining and being dissatisfied with what you've provided. Teach me meekness that I might praise you with all my heart. Thank you, Father, that I now can eat and be truly satisfied.

Yield to His Leading

Be ye not as the horse, or as the mule, which have no understanding: whose mouth must be held in with bit and bridle, lest they come near unto thee. Many sorrows shall be to the wicked: but he that trusteth in the Lord, mercy shall compass him about. (Ps. 32:9-10)

You know, a horse and a mule really have no understanding of where you want them to go or why, and so you use a bit and a bridle to control them and to get them to move where you want them (also to keep them from throwing you or biting you). But you know, they still are stubborn sometimes and won't go the way they should because they really aren't able to understand what you want them to do and why. David is saying to us not to be that way with God. We know we're on the road to thinness and temperance in eating. We know the way we must go to get there. Yet, we act like mules sometimes and make the Lord put a bit in our mouths even though it hurts more than just understanding and moving on.

God doesn't want to force us down the path to correct eating. If we yield to His leading He is merciful and will not allow it to be more painful for us than it has to be in order for us to learn. Remember, after our years of gluttony and overweight we deserve harshness from God, but instead he corrects us in love. Stop being a mule and walk on with God today, freely and with understanding.

Father, I'm sorry I've been a stubborn, fat mule, staying in the middle of the road and refusing to budge. You can take the bit and bridle off now because I'm ready to follow you. I know you are leading me on to a healthier, thinner, happier life and you're doing it because you love me. I also know that you will make the journey as painless as possible if I follow and accept the

44

necessary discomforts. I know I deserve harsh treatment, but your mercy has been shown to me and I thank you and praise you for all of this.

Your Deliverance

> The righteous cry, and the Lord heareth, and delivereth them out of all their troubles. The Lord is nigh unto them that are of a broken heart; and saveth such as be of a contrite spirit. Many are the afflictions of the righteous; but the Lord delivereth him out of them all. (Ps. 34:17-19)

If you are born again into the family of God through Jesus, then you are righteous in Him. God promises that He will hear you when you cry to Him. Perhaps you've fallen away from your diet or eating plan. Perhaps you never really began it in your heart and consequently were defeated. No matter why you're broken-hearted today, God is near and He hears if you come to Him in humility and repentance. He is faithful to forgive you and help you out of your situation. The Word says the righteous will have many trials, but that He will deliver us out of them all (not just some, all) if we are faithful to confess and repent.

Is your heart broken today because you've failed to do what God asked? Did you break your agreement with Him concerning your diet? Are you broken-hearted because you've never answered His call concerning eating habits? Well, call on Him now in humble repentance and obey whatever He tells you to do and He will deliver you from your situation and restore your joy!

Father, my heart is so heavy and I just can't go on this way. In Jesus' name, take this sin away. Thank you, Father, for I know I'm forgiven. Now reveal your will to me and lead me toward the eating schedule you would have me live on. Thank you again for your forgiveness and guidance.

Permanent Victory

> Rest in the Lord and wait patiently for him; fret not thyself because of him who prospereth in his way, because of the man who bringeth wicked devices to pass. (Ps. 37:7)

Many times we wait on God simply because we've done everything in ourselves that we could do. Then we turn to God and wait on Him for help. How many of man's diets have we used trying to lose weight or change our eating habits? How many of these have given us permanent results? God wants us to come to Him first with our problems and give them to Him so we can rest from the burden of them and wait on God's perfect solution. Take your eating problem to Him. If you have already, then just rest from it; quit struggling to work it out yourself because you can't. If you could have worked it out, you would have a long time ago, so admit you're helpless and let God carry the problem.

When God has worked His perfect work in you, you'll have a completely new eating life that will last a lifetime and will prolong that lifetime. Rest in the Lord, and He will truly bring it all to pass.

Lord, I know I keep trying to work it out myself and all I get is fatter and more frustrated. Take the problem of eating, Lord, and mold me completely to fit your perfect will. Instruct me and let me rest in the assurance that you know exactly what to do and that even now I am on my way to a new eating pattern. I ask this and thank you for it in the precious name of Jesus Christ.

If You Fall . . .

The steps of a good man are ordered by the Lord: and he delighteth in his way. Though he fall, he shall not be utterly cast down: for the Lord upholdeth him with his hand. (Ps. 37:23-24)

We can only be good through Jesus, who lives in us, and through allowing God to order our steps. When God is in control, our steps will be in the right direction and we will be happy in God's way because His way brings true happiness and peace.

So you were doing well on your diet? You were sure you had the problem licked and the old self under control. Then one day the old devil came along and tempted you, made you an offer of strawberry shortcake you couldn't refuse. You thought you could handle it and you were wrong. You fell and you fell hard, and the old devil got you on a self-condemnation trip. So now you feel everything is lost and God doesn't even want to hear from you anymore because you're so awful. Look at God's Word! It says that even if you fall, you won't be cast down by God. Instead, He is upholding you with His hand. One mistake and the loss of one battle doesn't mean you've lost the war. Remember God is the leader and He cannot lose the war if you give Him complete control and loyalty. So you fell. Pick yourself up, confess your sin to God and receive His forgiveness, then go on. Don't let Satan get you any further down; fight back. God is faithful to dust off your skinned knees and set you on your feet again. Look to Him and receive.

Father, forgive me for taking my eyes off you and yielding to temptation. Forgive me, in Jesus' name. I thank you for that forgiveness and ask that you set me on my feet again and strengthen me so I can go on. Thank you for the things I've learned, especially that I can always trust in you.

Confide in the Lord

But the salvation of the righteous is of the Lord: he is
their strength in the time of trouble. And the Lord shall
help them, and deliver them: he shall deliver them
from the wicked, and save them, because they trust in
him. (Ps. 37:39-40)

Have you noticed since you've been on a diet, losing weight
and having success in the Lord's plan, that some of your best
friends have become some of your worst enemies underneath?
Fatties and gluttons like to stick together to make themselves
feel better about what they're doing. When one of the "rank"
gets on God's bandwagon and starts walking in victory, the
others are envious of his success and inwardly disgusted with
themselves because they are still living the same old way and
waddling around fat. Sometimes the friendship is severed
completely, but many keep up the pretense of friendship and set
out to help you make the first fall. Then they can say, "I knew it
wouldn't work. There isn't any help for us." Now this may or
may not be a conscious effort, but either way the end result can
be the same if you fall for the bait.

The Word says your strength and salvation is in God. When
you're in trouble, call on Him. Don't go to a "friend" for help
when you're tempted. Most friends will convince you that one
little indiscretion is okay. But you'll hate yourself for it
afterwards. Go directly to God. He'll give you the correct
advice and the strength to carry out that advice. When you trust
in Him, He'll save you from the trap your "friends" set for you
and minister to them at the same time. They will see that God
has worked a miracle in your life and that there is hope for them
also. Trust in God no matter what He asks you to give up. He'll

48

give in return—something twice as good.

Father, I need your strength today. Make me strong in you so that I can resist whatever wrong food is offered me. Remind me that I must choose between you and the item tempting me, and I choose you. I trust in you to both deliver me and witness to my friends, who need your deliverance so much.

Hope in the Lord

Why art thou cast down, O my soul? and why art thou disquieted within me? hope thou in God: for I shall yet praise him, who is the health of my countenance, and my God. (Ps. 42:11)

Sometimes things go wrong during the day and we tend to forget from whom our health and strength comes. Perhaps the scales say you've gained a pound when you hope you had lost two. Perhaps you're feeling regret for that cookie you ate yesterday or even that extra salad you just had because it was allowed, not because you were hungry for it. If your soul is cast down, make Psalm 42:11 your cry unto God. Remind yourself that God is your hope and is responsible for your health and strength and for the forgiveness of your mistakes. Don't remain disquieted all day. Praise God no matter what your situation might be. He's still in power, still on His throne, so hope in His salvation and get happy!

I praise you, Father, just because I love you and because you've been so good to me. Oh, sweet heavenly Father, how precious you are to me. No matter what earthly matters seem like today, I want to rejoice in you because I trust and know that all is well. For you are both just and merciful.

Expectant Thanksgiving

Offer unto God thanksgiving; and pay thou vows unto
the most High: And call upon me in the day of trouble:
I will deliver thee, and thou shalt glorify me. (Ps.
50:14-15)

When we back ourselves into a corner by trying to fight our
own battles alone, it seems that we never fail to call on God for
help. Remember all the diets, fasting plans, and self-discipline
we tortured ourselves with before we finally fell before the Lord
in tears, asking for help? God wants us to come to Him first and
in a spirit of thanksgiving. When was the last time you really
thanked Him for what He has done and is doing to improve
your eating, nutrition, and to help you slim down? Do you thank
Him always or just when the scales say you've lost two pounds?
Do you only thank Him for what you can see has already
happened or do you thank Him in faith for what you know He
will do? You owe God your praise and thanksgiving each day.
His Word says if you've given this to Him as you should, then
when you call on Him for help, He'll give you that help—so you
will glorify Him. If you don't give Him thanks and glory in Him,
then you cannot claim the promise of His help in time of trouble,
because you aren't truly grateful. Praise Him for what He has
done, is doing, and will do in your life. Thank Him just because
you love Him, and He'll be near when you need Him.

Father, you've done so much for me. I could never fully
express my thanks and appreciation to you. Thank you for the
weight loss, the new eating plan, the discovery of your foods,
and the health you've given me. Thank you for what you're
doing right now in my body, soul, and spirit to change my life for
the better. Thank you for the discipline, weight loss, and food
plan I know you will give me in the future.

Justification from God

As for me, I will call upon God; and the Lord shall save me. Evening, and morning, at noon, will I pray, and cry aloud: and he shall hear my voice. He hath delivered my soul in peace from the battle that was against me: for there were many with me. (Ps. 55:16-18)

David is sorrowing that he has been reproached and buffeted by his friends and says he'll cry unto God. God delivers him in peace from the battle going on within as well as without. Sometimes it is hardest of all to take the rebuke of those that are closest to us, be it family or friends. When we've been following God and know His diet or eating plan is good and right, it's difficult, nevertheless, when well-meaning persons question us. They complain that we don't seem to be losing or that we aren't getting the proper nutrition. Others may take a stand by saying we've gone too far by applying religious convictions to eating habits or even that we're sinning by asking God for a better physical appearance. These things are hard to take without fighting back. But what does David say? Go to God with the situation. Call on Him for that inner peace you need to carry you through until the truth is visible to all.

Father, I've sought you and you answered me and gave me this new way of eating. You know what my [friends, family, etc.] are saying about it, and I can do nothing to change their minds. Teach me to love them through this and gently prove them wrong. Justify me, Lord, for I cannot justify myself. Give me peace and strength to go on even while everyone is against me because I am in your will.

The Holy Spirit Convicts

> Cast thy burden upon the Lord and he shall sustain
> thee: he shall never suffer the righteous to be moved.
> (Ps. 55:22)

Sometimes we have burdens we can't even try to carry
ourselves (and we really shouldn't because our Father is there to
take them for us). In David's case, he was asking God to defeat
his enemies. Perhaps your situation is different. Perhaps your
burden is trying to convince family members who do not have a
weight problem that they need God's good food as much as you
do. Perhaps they feel it's diet food and insist on eating the usual
junk foods that are slowly killing their bodies and causing you an
extra temptation. Maybe your burden is a family member or
friend who is a glutton, but not overweight, and just won't listen
to you or accept his sin. Whatever your burden, lay it before the
Lord and let Him carry it for you. You can't really help these
people anyway. Only the Holy Spirit can convict. All you can do
is yield the situation to God and let Him work out the best
solution for all concerned.

Lord, I just turn this situation over to you for your help and
guidance. Work it out and reveal your will to us all. We need
your help so badly. Use me to help in whatever way you will,
Lord.

Avoid Trouble

> Give us help from trouble: for vain is the help of man.
> (Ps. 60:11)

We've all called on God many times to help us when we were
in trouble, but here David asks God for help *from* trouble. We

know that we will always have troubles because we are tested and refined through our trials. But we can ask God for help from unnecessary trouble. There are troubles we can avoid. In our case, the trouble to avoid is poor health and fat bodies due to unhealthy eating habits. God's way of avoiding these troubles is perfect. He has provided, from the earth, foods good for our bodies. He dictates moderation in these. He advises us to avoid laziness, which causes flab. We have a right to call on God for this avoidance of trouble because it is His will for us to be healthy, and in good physical shape.

David says that man's help is vain. It isn't good enough and won't work. Look at all of the man-made food products we substitute for God's good, natural food. Every day we hear alarming statistics of how harmful these processed foods are and how little nutrition they actually contain. Many products are taken from the shelves because harmful chemicals have been used in the processing—chemicals that can cause disease and sometimes death. Seek God's help from trouble in eating. Follow His Word, not man's, and avoid health problems.

Father, help me steer clear of malnutrition, obesity and poor eating habits by revealing your Word concerning eating to me. I know I can remedy the trouble I'm in and avoid future dietary problems by following your Word and not man's devices and counterfeits. I ask and thank you, in Jesus' name.

Nothing is Hidden

O God, thou knowest my foolishness; and my sins are not hid from thee. (Ps. 69:5)

Have you ever felt like you could eat a cookie or have a few spoons of ice cream or whatever while you were home alone and that it wouldn't count? That's part of the "old self," isn't it?

It's funny how all those secret snacks become visible pounds on our fat bodies. Perhaps since you began this diet or eating plan, you've been stubborn about some food that you don't want to give up, so you pretend you haven't been convicted about it. Now you can fool family and friends; you might even fool yourself to a certain extent, but you can't fool God.

David said that God knew his foolishness and sin. God knows everything. You can't cheat Him behind His back; He knows. Yield today all that He has asked for and repent of your rebellion. Don't complain that God isn't working too well for you in dietary results when you've only yielded *some* to Him. Acknowledge your foolishness. He already knows about it anyway. Even if you're sure you've yielded all, go before Him and ask Him to expose your inner feelings and thoughts. You'll find He is constantly adding to and taking away from us in order to perfect us. You have nothing to lose and God's perfect will to gain, so do it now!

Father, I know that I can't hide anything from you because you know all things. Look into me, Lord, and reveal any sin or rebellion you see. Show me what I must do to make it right with you, and I yield myself to you to do it. Forgive my foolishness in Jesus' name.

Good Food

Who satisfieth thy mouth with good things; so that thy youth is renewed like the eagle's. (Ps. 103:5)

The average dieter would ignore the second half of this verse, and zero in on the first. It's that kind of thinking that will keep us in bondage all of our lives. The Scripture is God's Word and is true. Look at the "who" of the verse and consider this question. Are fatties ever satisfied? No! Do they have renewed youth and strength? Not usually. Then, apparently they've been looking to the wrong source for the good things for the mouth.

God is the true answer. He gives us good food—food that tastes good and is good for our physical bodies. The food He gives does satisfy because eaten temperately, it does not cause lustful craving. Because the food is good for us, it renews and restores our health and gives us new strength, so that we look and feel younger and stronger. It is God who supplies the good food to satisfy the body, and the same applies to His spiritual food.

Lord, I see it is your spiritual and physical food that satisfies and strengthens me. I turn my back on the bad and ask to be fed of the good, both physically and spiritually.

Sweet Words

How sweet are thy words unto my taste! Yea, sweeter than honey to my mouth! (Ps. 119:103)

Most people feel that verse of Psalm 119 is just a figure of speech, sort of an overstatement of the fact that God's words are good. When your stomach is aching and your spirit is longing, God's words can slip into you and you speak them and they satisfy and are more delicious than any gooey old dessert. Honey is concentrated sweetness, but God's Word will taste better and more satisfying than even honey. If you're in a slump today and are eating just to feel better or at least are tempted to do so, go before the Lord and start feasting on His Word (maybe through mealtime). Enjoy His delicacies and fill up on His promises and laws. See for yourself if His words are not sweeter than honey to your taste and more profitable than food to both your body and spirit. Your eating habit will take on a new meaning to you and victory will be yours!

Father, I have a banquet of your words before me to feast upon when I want, and I never realized it before. Lord, teach me to reach for your Word instead of the refrigerator. Let me hunger for your words of life, then fill me to overflowing with your truth that I might grow strong in spirit and temperate in the flesh.

Light in the Darkness

Thy word is a lamp unto my feet and a light unto my path. I have sworn, and I will perform it, that I will keep thy righteous judgments. (Ps. 119:105-106)

Anyone knows that if you walk around in the dark with no light to see where you are going, two things can and will happen. First, you'll end up a far piece from where you want to be, and second, you'll probably stumble and take a bad fall in the process (complete with bumps and bruises). This can happen to us when we're in the dark about diet and eating habits. Oh, we think we are well informed. After all, we've read every book ever written on the subject. But we are not slim for life as we want to be and have fallen so many times that even our bulges have bulges. But God's Word lets us see where we are going and all of the pitfalls along the way so we can avoid them if we wish to. Let's agree with God to keep His Word and His rules for diet and controlled eating. Stand firm and say, "I will do it in Jesus' name!"

Lord, my knees are tired of being skinned from all those falls, and my stomach just can't take another bulge. I give up! I've been groping in the dark for an answer that has always been available in your light. Light my path and lead me. I ask and pray this in Jesus' name.

Peace Through His Word

Great peace have they which love thy law: and nothing shall offend them. (Ps. 119:165)

If there's one thing that sounds good to a glutton, it is peace! With all the unrestrained eating to satisfy personal lust, compulsive eaters are never satisfied. Instead there is a driving force for more and more in an attempt to be satisfied and at peace, but somehow it never comes. All that results is anxiety over our fat bodies and our loathsome attitudes and a greater urge to eat—for comfort. What a vicious cycle, just filled with stumbling blocks!

God has given us the way out now, and we can eat well, eat less, and be at peace (which to some people sounds like agony and to others like a miracle). The Word says if we love His law (and therefore obey it) we will be at peace and there won't be any stumbling blocks in our way. This doesn't mean that we will literally not be tempted, but a stumbling block can only be a stumbling block when someone trips on it and falls. We will not trip and fall while walking in God's rules for diet and eating; we will be at peace.

Father, continue to show me your rules for diet and eating. Let me dwell in the peace of your will, for it is the only true and lasting peace there is. Expose those stumbling blocks to me as I approach them that I might leap over them in victory, not stumble and fall on them. Thank you, Lord, for your perfect will.

God is Not Silent

Behold, He that keepeth Israel shall neither slumber nor sleep. The Lord is thy keeper: the Lord is thy shade upon thy right hand. (Ps. 121:4-5)

Sometimes we find ourselves in the midst of an unforeseen trial or temptation and we feel so alone. It's as if Jesus and everyone in heaven was out to lunch somewhere and here we are, left alone to face our dilemma. Perhaps you were out shopping; a friend asked you over for lunch and you didn't see how you could refuse. When you got there, she gave you a choice of a salad or your favorite gooey dish from former days. You said, "Help, God! What should I do?" But there was only silence, so you thought God was busy elsewhere.

The Word says He doesn't sleep or slumber, even when you do. He is always there, always in control, always aware of everything that is happening. If you didn't get a reply from Him, maybe it's because He gave you the answer a long time ago. You see, there really was no decision for you to make. You had to choose the salad because the other dish was food you had already yielded to God, so it didn't belong to you. You created a problem for yourself by considering a sinful choice; therefore, you entertained the temptation and caused an emotional turmoil. Next time you don't hear God, remember what He has already said.

Father, thank you for all those moments of silence that say so much and lead me so beautifully and powerfully back on the right path. Thank you for being in control day and night. It is good to know that even when I'm asleep, you're not. You're right there watching over me and loving me.

His Strength Within Grows

In the day when I cried thou answeredst me, and strengthenedst me with strength in my soul. (Ps. 138:3)

David saw a truth in God that often we seem to miss or not acknowledge. When we're in a jam (that gooey dessert is staring us in the face), we know we aren't strong enough to resist by ourselves, so we scream to God for help and He hears us and gives us that extra strength to go on. But did you realize that it's a strength deep in the soul? It isn't just a shot of strength to get us through the next hour; it's a shot of long-lasting strength that remains with us if we'll acknowledge it. Each time God boosts us with strength in time of temptation, it increases His strength in our souls and makes the need for little shots fewer because we are using His built-in power source. The Spirit lives in you, and if you let Him control you totally, you will flow in His strength. The next time you need a shot of strength, be sure you claim a high-powered injection and grow in the Spirit.

Lord, it's so good to know you're there to strengthen me when I need it. I know now that each time you do, you add some built-in strength in my soul as I flow with your Spirit. Thank you so much for showing me this and for your Spirit within me.

Welcome the Trials

Though I walk in the midst of trouble, thou wilt revive me: thou shalt stretch forth thine hand against the wrath of mine enemies, and thy right hand shall save me. The Lord will perfect that which concerneth me: thy mercy, O Lord, endureth forever: forsake not the works of Thine own hands. (Ps. 138:7-8)

When you're in a mess, that's the time you really need to be looking in the correct direction for help. A time of deepest trouble can be a time of deepest peace and love between you and God if you are in harmony with God's Word concerning this situation. Perhaps you've reached a plateau in your diet where you don't seem to lose weight no matter how hard you try. Temptations to eat the wrong kind of foods have been too numerous to count. You've had a family crisis which tempts you to the old desire to eat for comfort, and you've got more work to do at home or on the job than ever.

It all sounds like too much, and you feel like you're drowning with no way of swimming to shore. Get happy and call on Jesus. He'll be right there to revive you if you turn it over to Him and trust Him for a miracle. The Word says God will protect you from the wrath of your enemies, and He's going to use temptation as a perfecting agent because you are His child and His creation. You can either trust God, look to Him for your answer and come out more like Him, or you can cry, scream, and try to get out of it your own way and come out spiritually weak and less perfect in the ways of God. The choice is yours. Choose God. With Him you'll never lose anything except the bad and never gain anything except the good.

Father, my life is in so much turmoil now that the bottom looks like up. I know there is no hope for my situation unless I turn it over to you. Take these circumstances and show me clearly what is necessary for me to do (or not to do) in each instance. Lord, I know you can turn this battle into a victory celebration, and I claim in Jesus' name, that it be so done. Thank you, Lord, for the answer.

Guard Your Mouth

Set a watch, O Lord, before my mouth; keep the door of my lips. (Ps. 141:3)

The power of the tongue or mouth is overlooked by so many Christians today, but for the dieter it is especially important to make Psalm 141:3 our daily prayer. The meaning of this verse is dual in nature. First, we want God to watch over our mouths, so we speak only good and edifying words. Often, by the confession of our mouth, we lose our victory in dieting or temperance. Such words like, "I can't resist," or "I just know I'll break," or "It's going to be so hard," or "I can't live without it," should be eliminated from our vocabulary before they wipe us out. The more negative your confession, the greater chance those bad things have of becoming a reality. So, the first part of the verse is about wrong speaking.

Second, the Lord needs to watch what goes into the door of our mouth. If we want the Lord's will in eating, then we need to have Him sound the alarm when we lift that bite of cheesecake to our lips. In verse four of Psalm 141, David comments on God not letting him eat the wrong food. We have a right to ask our Father to watch over us in this respect. God knows what food is bad and can give us discernment in our spirits that the food is wrong for us to eat.

Let God keep watch over your mouth and listen to His advice, because if you do, nothing bad will go in or out of your mouth and you will be in harmony with God's perfect will.

Father, I'm asking you to watch my mouth for me. I know that I don't always remember to be conscious of things that go in or come out, so I ask you to watch for me and remind me when I am out of line. Guide me in your perfect will.

The Lord Preserves

The Lord is righteous in all his ways, and holy is all his works. The Lord is nigh unto all that call upon him, to all that call upon him in truth. He will fulfil the desire of them that fear him: he also will hear their cry and will save them. The Lord preserveth all them that love him: but all the wicked will he destroy. My mouth shall speak the praise of the Lord: and let all flesh bless his holy name for ever and ever. (Ps. 145:17-21)

Did you ever accuse the Lord of not being fair? Well, you know He really isn't! That's right, nowhere does the Bible say that God is "fair"; it says He is righteous and just (among other things) but fair is a word that we've invented out of our selfishness. Fair is no substitute for justice or righteousness and we should be glad that it isn't one of God's terms. If God was "fair" with us (by our definition) we'd all have been annihilated a long time ago. God combines justice and mercy and so deals with us.

No matter what you *really* deserve today, if you need God and come to Him in a spirit of confession and repentance, He will be there. The Word says that if you call on Him in truth (you really mean what you ask), He'll hear and save you. If you've been on an eating binge, gained ten pounds and are distraught, that's a pretty legitimate time of need. Assuming you really want His help out of the whipped cream and cookies and into the clean path of His will, call to Him and His mercy will save you. If He were fair, He would leave you in your candy-coated mire, but He's merciful and will help you back to where you should be.

The Word says that God preserves us. Now everyone with a sweet tooth knows about "preserves." What are they? Usually fruit that has been prepared to keep a long time. Well, God preserves us; He keeps us from rotting and going bad. How sweet are His "preserves," His people!

Preserve me, Lord. Keep me in your protection. I strayed and missed the mark, but I'm back in truth, and desire the fulfilling sweetness of your way. Restore me, Father, in Jesus' name.

Healing the Broken Heart

He healeth the broken in heart, and bindeth up their wounds. (Ps. 147:3)

A broken heart can hurt more than physical pain sometimes and in the fleshly sense, there is no treatment for it. You can't soak it in hot water like a broken toe or bandage it like a cut or rub it like a strained muscle. All of us have experienced heartbreak and have soothed our wounds with food and junk food from time to time. Remember how little it really helped? In fact, it only made matters worse.

One thing that a glutton is broken-hearted over is being a glutton. One look in the mirror when dressing to go out or one look at the plate heaped with food the second time around is enough to break anyone's heart. I suppose in the back of our minds we think there is no help for this internal pain, so we turn to what we love best—food—for consolation and only increase the cause of our broken heart.

God can mend your heart, bind up those internal wounds and give you back your joy, peace, and health if you repent of your waywardness and turn to Him. If food is still your first love, your heart will still be broken. Give up that idol and worship only the Father. Then claim Psalm 147:3 and enjoy the miracle of God's love. When you are right with Him, He will heal your broken heart and take away the cause of it. Eating will never give you what you need.

Father, only you know what is in the depth of my heart. No one else can understand the reason my heart is broken, but you can. I turn to you confessing and repenting of using food (or whatever) for consolation and help. Take my fragile heart and mend and restore it that I might love you, others and myself as I should. Lord, I ask this in the name of Jesus Christ who shed His precious blood for me on the cross, that I might not have to suffer this broken heart.

The Promise of Wisdom

For the Lord giveth wisdom: out of his mouth cometh knowledge and understanding. He layeth up sound wisdom for the righteous: he is a buckler to them that walk uprightly. He keepeth the paths of judgment, and preserveth the way of his saints. (Prov. 2:6-8)

With all the *do's* and *don'ts* of sound nutrition today, perhaps you've had a hard time keeping straight what you should and shouldn't be eating or what is enough or too much of certain types of food. Maybe you're concerned you'll eat the wrong thing in your ignorance, and it will be harmful, not helpful, to your body. Well, that's possible, but God doesn't expect you to learn proper nutrition overnight either. The Word says that God has sound nutrition laid up for you. Go to His Word and search out what He has to say about food and nutrition. He promises knowledge and understanding, so ask Him when you don't know or aren't sure. Slowly He'll teach you the good and the bad foods and do the necessary weeding out in your eating. You are His saint and He promises to preserve your way if you walk in His way. That means He'll keep you safe and healthy if you are a good steward of your temple. So don't guess about nutrition. If you don't know about a food, look into the Word, and if it isn't found there, ask God to reveal to you His will concerning it.

Father, thank you for your Word concerning nutrition. Give me discernment. I know I have many years of misinformation to unlearn and lots of correct information to learn. Teach me, Lord, what I need to know that I might care for this temple properly in your eyes.

No Eating in Secret

Stolen waters are sweet and bread eaten in secret is pleasant. (Prov. 9:17)

When we sneak goodies they always taste better. An up-to-date writing of verse seventeen would be, "Snitched malts are even sweeter than those eaten when allowed and half a cake eaten behind everyone's back is so good." Of course, the reason for eating in secret is because we are ashamed; we know it's wrong and we shouldn't be doing it, but we just can't stand to hear anyone tell us so. We are not honest enough to do it in the open and stand up to the opposition, and do you know why? Because we know we are wrong and we would have to admit out loud that we do it out of our own selfish lust. We fear the conscious admission of the fact that we are gluttons. Somehow knowing it inside and saying it aloud are two different things.

Come out of the closets, bathrooms, carports, sheds, bedrooms (wherever it is you sneak off to eat) and face yourself. Go to a mirror and watch yourself eat that stolen food. See what everyone else has to look at when they watch you stuff your face full of food. Then say out loud to yourself, "I am a glutton and have sinned against God, myself and my family." Then seek forgiveness and do something about it.

Lord, forgive me for being a selfish glutton. Forgive all those sneaky snacks and stolen extra meals. Feed me on your Word and strengthen me with your discipline. From now on everything I eat will be in the open, so I might be a disciplined eater and show to those around me your power and glory. Should I be tempted to cheat, my family will know and help keep me straight. Thank you, Father, for showing me the truth about myself and giving me a change of heart.

No Escape from Discipline

Whoso loveth instruction loveth knowledge: but he that hateth reproof is brutish. (Prov. 12:1)

The word "instruction" can mean "teaching," but in a more concise rendering it means "discipline." Can we really love discipline? Of course, we can and do! Think of any hobby or project you've undertaken that you've wanted to excel in. You weren't looking for the fastest or easiest way out but the best way to achieve a perfect product. For instance, if you were making a patchwork quilt, you'd discipline yourself to take time and care with each stitch and redo each mistake. You wouldn't mind the redoing because you'd want a perfect quilt. Now the person who doesn't really care, who just wants a quilt to cover them, would either buy it ready-made or stitch it real fast and haphazardly on the machine and would learn very little about sewing or the art involved.

The person who is always looking for the easy way out will rarely learn to do anything right. The person who looks to the fastest diet, most closely related to his own eating desires (especially diets that encourage overeating) will never achieve permanent success, because he does not desire the knowledge of nutrition and weight control; he just wants quick and easy results. What he gets is a yo-yo weight-loss situation. But someone who wants to know and understand God's perfect will for nutrition and weight control will allow time and discipline to perfect body and spirit and turn out a beautiful product—a slim, fit, healthy body that will remain so the rest of his life. Discipline is good for you. Love it because it really pays.

Father, I don't want a sloppy body; I want that perfect finished product that only comes from long, careful days of learning and discipline. Teach me and mature me in your time and through your rules, and I know I will grow slim, strong, healthy, and warmly content in you.

To Be Satisfied

The righteous eateth to the satisfying of his soul: but the belly of the wicked shall want. (Prov. 13:25)

How many of us can say we are ever really satisfied with what we eat? How many times have you stuffed yourself and still wanted more because you lusted after the taste? There was no room in your stomach, so you had to stop. It's really sad to see someone get up from a table already fat, stuffed to capacity and still trying to get in one more bite as if food will go out of existence tomorrow. This is wicked, and because it is, the wicked person is not going to be satisfied. He will always want more. The more you lust after food, the more you will continue to lust and the less satisfied you will be.

He who is righteous follows God's method. One of God's basic rules on eating is temperance. Can you see why? Temperance just starves lust to death. A lustful appetite can't grow in the presence of temperance, so it dies. The dieter who is righteous with God in the area of food is not necessarily a person of great self-control, only a person yielded to following God no matter how long it takes. Such a person can sit down to fresh raw salad or cottage cheese and be satisfied. "Satisfying of his soul" is so descriptive of the truth. Your soul is the very part of you that is obedient to God, and when it is satisfied, you are truly content. Eat to take care of your bodily needs, not your fleshly lust.

How beautifully simple your Word is when the Spirit reveals it to us. For years I ate trying to satisfy my fleshly cravings; now I am satisfied in my soul and my flesh is silent because you have satisfied me completely. Thank you, Lord.

Your Response to Others

The eyes of the Lord are in every place, beholding the evil and the good. A wholesome tongue is a tree of life: but perverseness therein is a breach in the spirit. (Prov. 15:3-4)

Have you ever been caught eating a forbidden food? You know—the doorbell rings right in the middle of a piece of cake or something. What do you do? You try to stuff it in and swallow before you answer and you've got the guilty look of a murderer on your face by the time you reach the door. Then when you're confronted with the crumbs on your fat little chin, you become enraged at the intruders and treat them as if they are the ones caught doing something wrong. Or if a family member walks in when you're eating a one pound bag of M & M's and calls you on it, you really give them a tongue lashing. The Word says that speaking such bitterness and harshness breaks down your spirit and causes you even worse problems. If you're caught in the act, admit it! God probably arranged for it to happen to stop you from hurting yourself. The person is only trying to help you and you know it. It will go easier on you if you admit you blew it, ask forgiveness and tell that person you appreciate them. When you do, you will be speaking wholesome words that will benefit you spiritually and physically.

Father, I realize my mouth hasn't been speaking those things it should. Forgive me, in Jesus' name. Help me to realize and accept people's help. Keep me mindful of the fact that words are alive and can hurt or heal. Let me speak healing words to myself and others.

Seeds of Blessing

A man hath joy by the answer of his mouth: and a word spoken in due season, how good is it! (Prov. 15:23)

Have you ever noticed how excited a child gets when she has the right answer to a question in class? She'll just be bubbling with joy when she speaks it. That's the kind of joy we should have when we answer questions about our weight loss and change in eating habits. You should just get so excited about describing God's glory and power. When you do, you'll benefit from an inner joy that can't be explained.

Then, there are times when one of our fellow dieters is down or is having a battle with the devil and we've spoken just the right word that person needed to hear. For instance, a person feels like they aren't looking any thinner after a whole month of dieting, and you come along and tell them how much slimmer they look. How sweet those words are to that person and how uplifting.

We should do our best each day to speak good words to our friends and family, to uplift them and bring us personal joy. Sure, it is good when someone speaks that way to you, but if you want to reap good words spoken in due season, sow some yourself first. Be sensitive to the needs of others and you shall both bless and be blessed.

Thank you, Father, for giving me this means by which I can minister to others and bless them even as I am blessed. Help me to be sensitive to the needs of others and to meet their needs as best I can. I just bless you and love you, Lord.

Keep Your Walls Up

Hast thou found honey? eat so much as is sufficient for

thee, lest thou be filled therewith, and vomit it. . . . It is not good to eat much honey: so for men to search their own glory is not glory. He that hath no rule over his own spirit is like a city that is broken down and without walls. (Prov. 25:16, 27-28)

For some of us, the question about finding honey has a slightly different meaning. We can always buy it in a store. We don't usually stumble onto it in the field, but many of us are "finding" it for the first time. We were so used to refined sugar that we never thought of honey except for colds and occasionally on dinner rolls or biscuits. But now we know honey is a natural sweetener. The word of caution here is: don't overdo it. If you use honey as you did refined sugar, it's just as bad for you because your body can't take much. The Scripture says if you eat too much of it, you will get sick. Honey is twice as sweet as refined sugar, so use it sparingly.

On the spiritual level, seeking your own honor and glory and dwelling on your pride and the recognition you deserve is bad for you too. You'll get spiritually sick.

The last verse says you are weak and defenseless against the enemy if you don't have control over your body and spirit. If you are unrestrained and overindulgent physically with food, and emotionally with pride, you're as weak in spirit as a city without walls is in defense. The devil can step in and rip you apart because your walls are down.

Lord, through your Spirit I know I can exercise self-control and not be excessive in my life. Build up my body and spirit in you, that I might stand as a city with might, with high walls before Satan that he cannot prevail against.

Texture and Color, Aside

The full soul loatheth an honeycomb; but to the

hungry soul every bitter thing is sweet. (Prov. 27:7)

It's hard to believe that anyone would cast aside something sweet, but even a glutton reaches the point of having so much in his stomach that the thought of something sweet sickens him. A hungry person doesn't need something as rich as honeycomb to enjoy it; he'll eat anything that is set before him, and it tastes good.

Perhaps you now have better insight into what it means to be really hungry. We say we're hungry every day, but are we really hungry by scriptural definition? Will anything set before us satisfy us and taste good? No way! We're picky; we want variety and certain texture and color on our plate. We say we're hungry, but we only have a need to eat. When one is truly hungry, he'll eat what is available and enjoy it. So if you've been turning your nose up at some of God's good food, maybe you're still satiated with the old way of eating. Perhaps what you need is to fast before the Lord concerning your diet until even the most plain of God's good food looks like a feast.

Let go of your old tastes completely and hunger for God's food, which is good and satisfying. Hunger first, then He will fill and satisfy you. You can't hold on to old tastes and habits and expect new taste and habits to satisfy you. It won't work. Release the old and enjoy the new.

Father, I realize I don't know what hunger really is. I've spent so many years stuffing food in, I don't think my body has ever been allowed to be really hungry; therefore, I'm picky about food. Forgive me, Father. I release the old tastes to you and ask you to show me how to appreciate and be satisfied with the new.

Drugged by Food

For three things the earth is disquieted, and for four

which it cannot bear: For a servant when he reigneth; and a fool when he is filled with meat. . . . (Prov. 30:21-22)

One of the worst things that disquiets the earth or upsets nature is a fool when he's filled with meat. Why? Well, first of all, any glutton is a fool in respect to knowing how to care for himself. But it is unnatural to overeat. Our body was not meant to be overtaxed in that way, and the effect of overeating on the body is druglike. One becomes lazy, sleepy, and slow to move. What an abomination to see a fool stuffed with food, slumped in a chair, and stunned. It is as unnatural as a servant becoming king; it upsets the balance of nature.

Father, I'm your child and no fool. Teach me concerning foods and their effects on my body, that I might not upset the natural process you've ordained for my body when it is in top working order. I thank you and praise you for it in Jesus' name.

Idleness Can Breed Gluttony

She looketh well to the ways of her household, and eateth not the bread of idleness. (Prov. 31:27)

This Scripture is speaking of the virtuous woman but can apply to man or woman. This verse has a two-fold meaning. The first, of course, is the most obvious. The virtuous woman is one who takes care of her job and responsibility (in this case, at home, but it could be a career or whatever) and doesn't sit around idle all day watching TV, gossiping, napping, and neglecting work that needs to be done. In this respect, she doesn't eat the bread of idleness.

The deeper significance is that the "bread of idleness" can be literal food. Yes, we know it's true that munching and snacking all day can be due to idleness. We sit around and the less we do, the less we care to do, and the whole day becomes a series of eating spells from one snack to another until we go to bed. This is one important reason for staying healthy and productive. If you're not sitting around bored with nothing to do, you aren't as open to the devil's temptation of food. Get out and do something for God, your family, your friends. Be productive; get a job if you really have nothing to do at home. If you sit home idle, you'll reap the bread of idleness two-fold.

Father, I want to be virtuous, not bored or idle. Show me projects and jobs that I can do to use time wisely. Teach me how to do things for family and friends and where I can actively work for you. I'm tired of snacking my life away and feeling so fat and unproductive. I want to work for you now so show me how.

From the Hand of God

> There is nothing better for a man, than that he should eat and drink, and that he should make his soul enjoy good in his labour. This also I saw, that it was from the hand of God. (Eccles. 2:24)

There's nothing more satisfying to a person than putting food on the table which has been earned through honest work. It's a good feeling to know you've worked and earned the money to provide food and other necessities for your family. It is God's desire that you enjoy this food. That's right, God wants you to enjoy food and eating. He wants it to be a pleasant experience. This is one of the pleasures of life He desires for His children.

But you can't really enjoy food and drink without God. There's your limitation on quality and quantity. Surely, God wants you to enjoy His good food that is pleasant to taste and healthy for the body. When you sit at the table to eat and you offer a prayer of thanksgiving to God for the food, how can you ask Him to bless foods that will harm you? He cannot do it; it is contrary to His will and His whole being. Do you ever ask God to bless the food to His use? How can you do that with a straight face knowing the food is of poor quality and as soon as the prayer is finished you intend to stuff yourself full to overflowing? Enjoy the fruit of your labor—but with God's limit—and be pleased in your soul.

Father, I am thankful for the food you allow me to earn by my labor. I am grateful that you meant for eating to be a pleasurable experience. There's no pleasure in the way my stomach feels when I've overeaten and abused my body with the wrong foods. Lord, if there is a food offensive to you on my table, when I ask the blessing, point out that food that we might not partake of it but eat only that which is blessed of you.

Patience and Trust

Better is the end of a thing than the beginning thereof: and the patient in spirit is better than the proud in spirit. (Eccles. 7:8)

It's no simple thing to turn your life around and go with God. There are so many pressures from within and without and at first, it seems like such a long, hard road to reach the point of really eating and living as God will. Sometimes you think, "I can do this now while I'm losing weight, but can I really grow to the point of enjoying this as a way of life?" This is where trusting God for a miracle comes into play. If you have faith in God, He will not only change your outward appearance, He'll change your inward attitudes. At the beginning it's sometimes hard to see all of that. The patient person is the wise one. The one who has faith in God's ability (not his own) to change him and who hangs in there and goes on is the one who receives the reward of victory. Even though it's painful in the beginning, at the end of a diet, you are slim, trim, and healthy outside and you are temperate and spiritually mature on the inside because you believed God.

Now the person who is proud and arrogant about the diet, trusting in his will power and ability (instead of patiently waiting on God and walking in His care) will not reach a peaceful end because he does not acknowledge the source of success: God! Be wise by being patient and win the prize God gives.

Father, it seems hard now and I can't see yet all you're trying to teach me and show me. I have a long way to go and even though I don't move as fast as I want to, I know you are in control. I believe you, Lord. I trust and know you will bring me to a victorious end in your perfect time. Thank you and praise you, Lord!

He Will Forgive You

Come now, and let us reason together, saith the Lord: though your sins be as scarlet, they shall be as white as snow; though they be red like crimson, they shall be as wool. (Isa. 1:18)

One of the devil's favorite tricks to defeat the Christian is condemnation and guilt. If you are having a problem forgiving yourself or believing God could forgive you, you can be set free today.

Dieters especially seem to have trouble forgiving themselves when they cheat. You think, "God has been so good to me. I promised not to eat candy again, and here I sit with an empty one pound bag of M & M's. How can He forgive me?"

We are not strangers to God. He's our Father, and He says we

out together. Even if you're so steeped in sin
...carlet, He is *willing* and *able* to wash you white
...esn't matter what you've done; if you confess and
...pent in Jesus' name, it is His will and desire to forgive you, and
He is faithful to do so.

Don't let the devil or anyone else keep you in
self-condemnation or uncertainty concerning God's
forgiveness. He forgives you, and you must forgive yourself.

Father, forgive me for being so foolish. You know what I've
done and how sorry I am. I confess in Jesus' name and ask to be
forgiven. Thank you for the forgiveness and for helping me to
forgive myself.

Meditate on God

> Thou wilt keep him in perfect peace, whose mind is
> stayed on thee: because he trusteth in thee. Trust ye in
> the Lord for ever: for in the Lord Jehovah is
> everlasting strength. (Isa. 26:3-4)

Many people have excuses as to why they won't go on a diet
or why they can't give up white flour and refined sugar. When
God has revealed His word concerning food and eating to
someone, there's no excuse as to why it won't work for them
and why they can't do what He asks. The basic argument is that
giving up the most loved foods permanently would cause a daily
mental and physical anguish that would make life unbearable.
Also, cutting back on quantities would leave one always hungry
and physically uncomfortable. Well, in the natural sense, this
sounds logical, but it is not so with God. You see, God is the one
big factor that makes the difference. Proper eating without God
might do all the above mentioned, but when God is the
motivating and altering factor, it's a whole different situation.

The Word says if you are trusting God, depending on Him,

and keeping your mind stayed on Him, He'll give you perfect peace. When God says "perfect," He means just that. He will provide the peace, and as your obedience grows, He'll remove the unpleasant physical feelings and replace them with a satisfaction you never knew before. He will give you the strength as long as your eyes are on Him because He is the source of strength, not your own will power or self-discipline.

If you're on a diet and feel a little weak or lost, look to God. Get your eyes back on Him and enter into His peace. Be strengthened in your resolve as you draw close to Him. With God, there is no such thing as failure, only success. Give Him a chance to prove to you His word is true. Trust Him!

Father, I'm putting myself in your hands and fixing my eyes firmly on you. I trust you to keep me in peace and strength as long as I am looking to you and leaning on your power and strength. I thank you, Father, for peace and strength.

A Time for Variety

Doth the plowman plow all day to sow? Doth he open and break the clods of his ground? When he hath made plain the face thereof, doth he not cast abroad the fitches, and scatter the cummin, and cast in the principal wheat and the appointed barley and the rie in their place? For his God doth instruct him to discretion, and doth teach him. (Isa. 28:24-26)

The significant point here is that God is the great teacher (if we will be teachable) in every area of life. A farmer who wants to plant doesn't continue to plow all the time. He plows, then plants his various grains in their proper place. God shows him how to do these things and when.

We dieters can tap into God's teaching power also. We won't be losing weight always and won't be eliminating certain foods on a permanent basis. Sure there are foods—the weeds and stones in the field—that have to go completely. But some foods only need to be taken away for a while. For instance, when plowing a field, all plants and vegetation have to go, but when the planting is done, then the good plants are allowed to grow and remain. Our eating is the same. We have to sow good food in our eating plan, and once we're slim, we can allow all good food in our field. God will instruct us in due season. He will tell us what to weed out and what to plant. He'll show us what we can add to our diet and when the perfect time to add it is. What a wonderful teacher the Lord is!

Lord, teach me to plow up my diet and weed out all the harmful foods. Then let me plant the seed of good food in my body that I might grow slim and strong. Add and subtract foods as you see fit and as is good for me, Lord. Teach me daily to be discriminate concerning my diet.

God Gives Victory

It shall even be as when an hungry man dreameth, and behold, he eateth; but he awaketh, and his soul is empty; or as when a thirsty man dreameth, and behold, he drinketh; but he awaketh and behold, he is faint, and his soul hath appetite: so shall the multitude of all the nations be, that fight against Mount Zion. (Isa. 29:8)

The Lord speaks here of the victory of Jerusalem and how her enemies will dream of victory over her, but when they wake it will not be so. They will be defeated and will not win over Jerusalem.

Many of us experience a similar situation in two ways. First, when we begin a diet, usually we experience hunger and often dream of eating our favorite foods. Of course, when we awake it all vanishes and we are still hungry. On a deeper level however, we experience this when we diet in our own strength without God's help and outside of His perfect plan. We daydream and dream about the victory over that fat and gluttony, but that's all it is—just a dream. Any success is limited, the war is never won. Soon we begin to believe all it could ever be is a dream. Year after year we dream of being thin and energetic, eating and enjoying healthy food, but our bodies aren't impressed by that dream. But God can and does change that. He's on our side and can make our good dreams of fitness come true and make that nightmare of our life just a bad dream. Why not wake up to a dream-come-true in Jesus today.

Lord, for years I've dreamed of being thin and a healthy eater. I ask in Jesus' name that you make that dream a reality. I yield to your will and accept the victory as you instruct me.

Just Hang On

Say to them that are of a fearful heart, Be strong, fear not: behold, your God will come with vengeance, even God with a recompence; he will come and save you. (Isa. 35:4)

The Lord was encouraging His people with prophecy of the return to Zion when all would be well with His people and they would dwell in safety and happiness. Jesus has come and we can have the fulfillment of these words within our lives because Jesus lives within us.

It seems just when your new way of eating is really going along smoothly and temptation is almost a thing of the past, that the old devil tries to stop you. All of a sudden, problems seem to be coming from every direction (you know, the kind that used to drive you to the cookie jar or refrigerator). Even as you resist the urge to eat for consolation, behold, your weight loss seems to stop for no real reason, or you even gain a pound or two. Now if you still don't fall, the old devil begins to put doubts and fears in your head concerning your eating. He tells you maybe you blew it somehow and God is punishing you, or perhaps you've lost all you can or will lose. At this point, you can do one of two things. Either you give in to the devil and blow it, or you can get happy, and praise God for the exciting miracle He's about to work. You know, God doesn't ever ask or tell us to do anything unless He knows we can. Therefore, when He says to be strong and not fear, He knows we can do it because we are in Him. If you've reached the point of blowing it, just hang on because God will come to your rescue, work a miracle or two, and send the old devil running. Trust God for that miracle. He will not fail you.

Father, you know that every direction I look there's another battle to be fought. I'm surrounded by the enemy, Lord, and he's closing in, but I'm getting happy because I know I'm in miracle land. There's no way out for me in earthly ways, so I know I'm in line for a miracle from you. Come to my aid, Lord. Strengthen me and save me.

Promise of Deliverance

Fear thou not; for I am with thee; be not dismayed; for I am thy God: I will strengthen thee; yea, I will help thee; yea, I will uphold thee with the right hand of my righteousness. (Isa. 41:10)

God is speaking to Israel here and promising to be with her and uphold her always. We are grafted-in children of Abraham and, therefore, part of the descendants of Jacob and heirs to this promise. This is a precious promise that assures us that God is always there and on our side as we stay in His will.

Perhaps that first really big test is soon approaching. You've confessed God's power in your changed life and eating habits. You've been firm month after month about not eating sugar or refined flour or whatever God has removed from your life. You're looking and feeling great; you've just arrived at your desired weight, and things are wonderful. But it's vacation time, and you're going on a family trip. Perhaps you fear your vacation because of the old attitude of "food" and "fun" being synonymous. Maybe you're going to be visiting a family that cooks nutritionally poor foods and has lots of your old favorite junk foods. This may even be an eating binge you formerly looked forward to every year. Whatever the case, you're afraid you'll blow it after all this time.

Begin claiming Isaiah 41:10. Be conscious of the fact that God is with you. When a situation begins to look difficult, don't let it worry you, for God says He will give you the strength you need just at the right time. He will uplift you and give you victory if you look to Him and listen to His commandments. Turn that trip into a pilgrimage of victory for the Lord!

Father, you know what lies ahead for me on this trip. Be with me at all times watching for any holes I might fall into or stumbling blocks I might trip over. Give me strength when I need it and protection. I ask and pray in Jesus' name with praise and thanksgiving for the victory.

Trials for Our Perfection

But now thus saith the Lord that created thee, O Jacob, and he that formed thee, O Israel, Fear not: for I have redeemed thee, I have called thee by thy name; thou art mine. When thou passest through the waters, I will be with thee; and through the rivers, they shall not overflow thee: when thou walkest through the fire, thou shall not be burned; neither shall the flame kindle upon thee. (Isa. 43:1-2)

Although we can depend on God to strengthen us and give us the ability to resist temptation, that does not mean we will not have trials, tests, and hard times. We are in the world and God allows us to face trials to help us mature. The assurance He does give is that He'll be right there with us and, if we look to Him in trust, He will not allow any harm to come to us.

God doesn't guarantee you'll never have another hunger pang if you diet His way, nor does He insure you'll never face a chance to be gluttonous. On the contrary, these things must come in order to strengthen us. Think of each trial as a final exam in that area. If you pass with flying colors, you'll be promoted and not have to keep taking the same test over. You graduate and move on.

Look to God. Lean on Him and depend on Him for strength. Face the trials and go through them with Him. Don't think He'll skip you over them; He never promised that. He said He'd go through them with you and He will, and you'll come out together on the hallelujah side.

Father, I know trials must come to strengthen me, but as long as you are with me, I know I can go through them in strength and faith. Make me thankful for the trials, Lord, because I know it is for my perfecting.

Healed of Gluttony

But he was wounded for our transgressions, he was bruised for our iniquities: the chastisement of our peace was upon him; and with his stripes we are healed. (Isa. 53:5)

In most cases, obesity is a sickness, and it in turn causes diverse sicknesses. In some cases, deliverance is needed, but in all, God's healing is needed. How do we know if God wants us healed? Of course, simple logic tells us that if the Word of God is true and God loves us as He says He does, then He doesn't want us sick and suffering. Jesus bore all our sickness and disease, so we wouldn't have to be sick. The Word says we "are healed"; that's past tense—not we *could* be healed or *maybe* will be healed, but we *are*.

If you've put off asking God to heal you of your eating problem, don't wait any longer. It is God's good pleasure to heal you, and He desires to do so. Why pay a debt twice on purpose? Jesus paid the cost for you; don't pay it again by accepting sickness. Refuse it in Jesus' name.

Father, thank you for sending Jesus to save us all from the eternal fire and from the world. Thank you for loving us so, Jesus, that you bore our sins and sicknesses on the cross that we might have a free and abundant life here on earth. I thank and praise you, Lord.

God's Word is Faithful

So shall my word be that goeth forth out of my mouth: it shall not return unto me void, but it shall accomplish that which I please, and it shall prosper in the thing whereto I send it. (Isa. 55:11)

We all have a bad habit of speaking idle words. Sometimes it's just to make small talk. Other times we make commitments and promises we don't keep because we didn't give thought to what we said. God is not that way. He does not speak idle words but is faithful to accomplish those things His words say. God's words are spirit and are alive, and His Word says they will accomplish what they're sent to do. By all means, do what He says, for you are assured of the promised results. If you see a promise written in the Bible, claim it and you shall have it.

God is faithful. He never goes back on His Word even when we don't deserve His faithfulness. As you read the Bible and learn about foods and eating patterns, listen to the Word and act accordingly, and you shall have the body and health you desire.

Thank you, Father, for showing me your will and so many promises concerning eating. I am more than grateful that you do not speak idle words because I know when you speak, you will do what you say. Thank you, Lord.

Give of Your Food

Is it not to deal thy bread to the hungry, and that thou bring the poor that are cast out to thy house? when thou seest the naked, that thou cover him; and that thou hide not thyself from thine own flesh? (Isa. 58:7)

If there is one thing that comes hard, it's learning to give up food. Yet God says one of the aspects of an acceptable fast is to share food with the hungry. When was the last time you shared food? Perhaps your diet is not going as well as it should be because you are still selfish about "your" food. Why not break free of that bondage and fast, giving to a needy cause the money you would have spent on food that day.

You are also to help the needy and not run when a relative needs help. If it sounds like a hard road, think of all Jesus gave up for you. It's a small sacrifice in light of all Jesus went through. Learn to put yourself last (especially concerning food) and begin to enjoy the freedom of no longer being bound by eating.

Teach me, Father, to share and give freely to others all that I have, especially food. I want to help others, to feed those who have no food from the abundance I have. Teach me to die to self in this, Lord.

There Are Others

Thy words were found, and I did eat them; and thy word was unto me the joy and rejoicing of mine heart: for I am called by thy name, O Lord God of hosts. (Jer. 15:16)

Jeremiah was complaining to the Lord and reminding God of all the persecution he was going through for God, and blamed God for not stopping the people from hurting Him. He spoke the words of verse sixteen to God, but proceeded to say God was undependable and unpredictable. Does this sound familiar?

We've been on a diet for a month or so, and first thing you know, everyone around us is trying to tell us different things to do or not do; temptations are coming from every direction. Sometimes we hear God and sometimes we don't, but we testify outwardly that God's Word is a joy to us and we are so glad we are His. Then we go to God and say, "You've failed me. You led me into this and now I'm the only one. Even my friends think I'm fanatic."

Chances are God will say to you the same as He did to Jeremiah. "Stop being a fool and listen to me. Unless you yield to me and do as I say, you can't walk and talk for me." God showed Jeremiah he wasn't alone, that He had reserved a whole group of people to himself. If you will trust God, He'll reveal others to you whom He has called in this area.

When you say you rejoice in God's Word and are really glad and proud to be called by His name, mean it. If you attach any qualifications to it, don't say it. God is faithful. He is not inconstant nor is He negligent. Be patient and He will work in His perfect time.

Father, thank you for the privilege of standing for you even in the face of opposition and criticism. It is enough for me to stand for you and rejoice in the promises of your word as your child. I thank you and praise you in Jesus' precious name.

God is Not Fooled

The heart is deceitful above all things, and desperately wicked: who can know it? I the Lord search the heart, I try the reins, even to give every man according to his ways, and according to the fruit of his doings. (Jer. 17:9-10)

In the world we can lie and cheat people because they don't know any better. We can tell a person we love them and look so convincing and they'll believe us whether it's really true or not. No one but God knows what's really in our hearts, and we can't lie to Him, even though we often try.

How many times have you told God and others you really want to give up your gluttony? How many times have you tried to say, "I really don't eat that much. I don't understand why I gain weight"? Or how about "I've been faithful to my diet and I just can't lose; in fact I gained two pounds." You might fool others and even yourself, but you can't fool God.

The Word says God knows what's really in your heart. He tries you and lets you go in your own way if you choose, but there's a price! You can't expect to satisfy your own selfish appetite and get the same results as one yielded to God's way of eating. It just doesn't happen.

Face yourself today. Check your motives, write down

everything you eat, even any taste you might take; measure—don't estimate—quantities, and see if you are really adhering to your diet.

Father, I realize I've been stubborn and selfish. Forgive me, in Jesus' name. Show me where I've cheated and what I've done wrong so I can change and achieve proper results. I'll be honest with you, Lord. You know my very deepest thoughts. Thank you for showing me my faults and setting me straight.

Devour God's Word

Moreover he said unto me, Son of man, eat that thou findest; eat this roll, and go speak unto the house of Israel. So I opened my mouth, and he caused me to eat that roll. And he said unto me, Son of man, cause thy belly to eat, and fill thy bowels with this roll that I give thee. Then did I eat it; and it was in my mouth as honey for sweetness. (Ezek. 3:1-3)

It wasn't a dinner roll God gave Ezekiel to eat; it was a scroll with God's Word on it. God was impressing Ezekiel with the importance of getting God's Word chewed and digested, so it could nourish and become itself a part of him. God's Word should be sweet to our taste for it is truth. Whenever God's Word tastes bitter to us, it is not His Word but the bitterness of rebellion that we taste.

Have you found God's Word concerning diet and eating habits harsh, bitter, hard to swallow? Then the trouble is in you, not in His Word. Read the Bible, meditate on it, chew it, swallow it, and let it fill you completely. Yield to it and taste its sweetness, not in your mouth but your soul. Can honey ever be bitter? God's Word is the same way; it can never be bitter. Only your refusal to yield to it causes bitterness.

Father, teach me to feast upon your Word and savor every paragraph and sentence. Fill my insides with the sweetness and goodness of your Word that I might be able to speak it in faith and power to others who need it.

Food that Defiles

> And the king appointed them a daily provision of the king's meat, and of the wine which he drank. . . . But Daniel purposed in his heart that he would not defile himself with the portion of the king's meat, nor with the wine which he drank. (Dan. 1:5, 8)

Daniel was a captive of Nebuchadnezzar and was one of the youths chosen for training to become a counselor to the king. Now the king wanted these men to be strong and healthy, so he appointed them the best food from his own kitchen. Who wouldn't jump at a chance like that? Daniel wouldn't! Why? Because he didn't want to defile himself with nonkosher food, food which God said was bad for him.

The man in charge of Daniel was afraid to let him eat other food because he was concerned Daniel's health would be affected adversely. But Daniel knew you can't lose with God, and he proved it to this servant of the king. He and his men ate only as God allowed. After ten days they looked healthier than the rest, so they were granted permission to stay on their diet.

It would have been so simple for Daniel to cop out by saying, "Well, I'm a prisoner and have to eat what I'm told." Sure, he was probably tempted by the rich food of the king, but he knew he had to request other food rather than defile his body, even if it meant death for refusing the king.

How often have you taken the easy way out and eaten what you shouldn't have just because it was placed before you? How many times have you not spoken up, but have silently eaten forbidden food? There is no need to step out of His will by eating the wrong foods. Stand as Daniel did. Don't let anyone make you concerned for your health. Quite the contrary, you've been eating unhealthy foods all your life. Now that you're eating God's way you can't help but have improved health.

Father, be with me each time the "dainties of the king" are placed before me. Strengthen me that I might speak up and refuse them, not pridefully, but humbly and with grace. Make an avenue, so I can receive acceptable food and never be forced to eat the wrong food. Make me aware of the fact that, if I eat wrong food, it is by choice, not necessity. I pray and thank you in Jesus' name.

A Ten-Day Trial

Prove thy servants, I beseech thee, ten days; and let them give us pulse to eat, and water to drink. (Dan 1:12)

Again we refer to Daniel and his ten-day diet. Here we concentrate on the fact that he asked for vegetables and water only. Now this probably also included grains and grain products, so Daniel and his companions were only eliminating meat and strong drink. They did receive protein from the food they ate because the grains and vegetables were unprocessed and unrefined. (Vegetarians today have a harder time getting their proper protein in its best form.) After ten days, the Scripture says they looked so great that the diet was continued.

No matter what diet God calls you to, it will be good for you, and He will bless you in it. Perhaps you'd like to give His eating plan a ten-day trial, and then when you see the results, you can put your whole family on it for good health. Seek God concerning proper eating for you. It may be vegetarian or carnivorous, but God will be sure it is best for you.

Daniel chose to eat what was good for him, not what might have seemed good to him. We should apply that same wisdom to our lives in all areas but especially in food and nutrition.

Father, I'll give you a try. You tell me what I should and shouldn't eat and I'll try it for ten days. If I'm healthier and slimmer in ten days, I'll stick with it, change my eating, and attempt to change my family's eating also, that we might all be healthy and strong. I ask in Jesus' name, and I thank you for the results.

Playing the Harlot

> For their mother hath played the harlot: she that conceived them hath done shamefully: for she said, I will go after my lovers, that give me my bread and my water, my wool and my flax, mine oil and my drink. (Hos. 2:5)

The "mother" in this Scripture has a dual reference; it speaks of both Israel as a nation and Hosea's wife in the flesh. The Lord, in speaking to Hosea, compared Israel (Hosea's wife) to a harlot who leaves her home, husband and children to seek her lovers. But why does she run after her lovers? Because they give her food, drink, and clothing that she delights in. Apparently, she esteems these things more than the love of her husband and family. God was saying here that Israel was seeking her lovers, her other gods, because they fed and satisfied her appetites and gave her what she selfishly wanted.

Who do you love today, dieter? Do you love Jesus? Do you love food? Do you love a certain diet because you can have lots of meat and cheese and stuff yourself? Have you been playing the harlot in your heart, running after your appetite and the fulfillment of your lust for food, and leaving the Lord behind? Think about it! Have you been doing this? If so, you need to turn around and head back in the right direction.

Father, I repent of my sin. Forgive me in Jesus' name for playing the harlot with diets and people who feed my food desires. Take me back and restore your covering upon me.

Not by Bread Alone

> But he answered and said, It is written, Man shall not live by bread alone, but by every word that proceedeth out of the mouth of God. (Matt. 4:4)

It is a fact that without food, the human body cannot continue to exist. If the body goes for too long without food, it dies. Jesus did not presume to disagree with this known fact, but He did assure us in Matthew 4:4 that just food can't keep a person "alive."

"Well, what about the atheist?" you say. "They don't acknowledge God's Word, yet they continue to live on mere food!" No, they don't! The "life" Jesus was speaking of was true life, the life of the spirit, not just the body. No amount of physical food can keep you alive and healthy in spirit. Only feeding on God's Word can sustain the spirit and keep it healthy and growing.

As we diet, we can stand on these words of Jesus. The good food we eat will keep our bodies healthy and strong, but God's Word will build up our spirits that we might be able to speak God's Word with authority and stand fast in our new way of physical eating. Perhaps the pick-me-up we need for our eating plan isn't more variety in physical food but a refreshing variety of God's spiritual food. Let's try it today!

Lord, I know that if physical food could give life, I'd be more than alive; but only your Word can really build me up in spirit and keep me eating right for my body. Feed me on your Word, the words of your mouth, because they are spirit, they are life. Thank you, Father, for your words and your leading.

First Things First

> But seek ye first the kingdom of God, and his righteousness; and all these things shall be added unto you. (Matt: 6:33)

Jesus was admonishing His followers not to be concerned about the necessities of life (i.e., food, clothing, shelter) because they are not as important as seeking the living God and His kingdom. He tells them that God knows they need these things and that, if they put Him first, He'll give them their needs.

Sometimes we get so caught up in trying to eat right and control our weight and appetite that we become anxious about these things and mess up our list of priorities. God knows that we desire to eat well and temperately and He will provide the necessary food and knowledge in due time. It is more important that we seek the Lord and spiritual growth in all areas first; then He will meet our physical needs.

Have you spent more time reading nutrition and diet books than the Word of God? Can you quote Linda Clark, chapter and verse, better than you can quote Jesus? If the answer is yes, your priorities are out of line and you are too caught up with worldly cares. Yes, God wants you to be temperate and knowledgable about nutrition, but He first wants you to have a right relationship with Him and spiritual growth. When you put these first in your life, He will make provision for the rest of your temporal needs. Try Him and see that He is faithful to do what He has said.

I know that sometimes I get so caught up in my crusade for nutritious eating and weight control that I get ahead of myself and forget the source of my strength and freedom. Forgive me, in Jesus' name, Father. Set my priorities straight and lead me in your ways. I know as I grow in you and in your Word, that you will provide for my dietary and weight loss needs.

Expect an Answer

Ask, and it shall be given you; seek, and ye shall find; knock, and it shall be opened unto you. (Matt. 7:7)

Our heavenly Father is so merciful to us, yet we still underestimate Him sometimes. We think we are the exception, we are the case that's just a little too tough for God to handle. There is no problem so great that God can't solve it if we give Him full control of the situation. Even if it is a lifelong problem like compulsive eating, gluttony, overweight, etc., God can and will deliver us if we ask.

"I asked," you say, "but nothing happened." Now either you or God is a liar because the Word says if you ask, you'll receive. Of course, you must ask in His will, but we already know it is His will to set you free of fat and poor eating habits. "Then what did I do wrong?" Nothing; you have yielded and asked, so thank Him, sit back, and wait for your help because the Word says you will have it. If you need knowledge concerning God's plan for you, keep seeking and you will find. You have God's word on it and you can't get any better than that!

Lord, thank you for showing me in your Word that I will

receive the answer to my prayer of need. I know I'm in your will. I've asked in Jesus' name, and now I'm awaiting my answer in praise and thanksgiving. Praise you, Father, that your promises are true and for today.

Die to Self

He that findeth his life shall lose it: and he that loseth his life for my sake shall find it. (Matt. 10:39)

On the surface, Jesus seems to be doing some double-talk here, but when we look closer, we see the deeper meaning of His words. He is saying that if we hold on to our lower, fleshly life, we'll lose our higher spiritual life. On the other hand, if we are willing to give up our lower life, then we will have the higher life.

Of course, the Lord wants us to enjoy the things of the earth while we are here, but where do our love and commitment lie? If we seek after the pleasures and desires of the flesh, like food and fleshly appetite, and this is our main goal in life, we cannot attain the higher, spiritual life.

By choosing our new eating habits and weight loss program, we are saying in a practical way that we choose the higher life. We seek after the eternal and lasting life in Jesus. This is our goal—not slavery to the flesh. We must die to self in order that we might live for Him. If you haven't died yet, do it today. It's your privilege.

Father, you know how earthly things get me so trapped sometimes. All my life I've lived to eat and never was I really alive. Now I'm alive in you and I thank you that I now eat to live. Teach me how to continue to die to self that I might live in you.

A Much Lighter Yoke

Come unto me, all ye that labour and are heavy laden, and I will give you rest. Take my yoke upon you, and learn of me; for I am meek and lowly in heart: and ye shall find rest unto your souls. For my yoke is easy, and my burden is light. (Matt. 11:28-30)

Have you ever been burdened? Of course you have; everyone has. The compulsive eater especially knows what it's like; food is the heavy burden we bear. The yoke of that burden was harsh and harmful, physically and emotionally painful. It always seemed like it would never end, and freedom was nowhere in sight. But then Jesus stepped in and rescued us.

The yoke of gluttony and compulsive eating was not something we consciously asked for. The devil tempted us, laid it on us, and we thought we were stuck with it. The Lord's yoke is different; it is a chosen yoke which Jesus says is not harsh or painful, but pleasant. His burden is light. By choosing His yoke we choose peace and freedom in Him.

Every born-again believer has a right as part of his inheritance to take on the yoke of Jesus. In fact, it not only is a right but a necessity if we're to grow in Him. Therein lies the peace each of us had sought for so long but never could find. There is the happiness the glutton never could know, and there is the key to temperance which sets us free.

Lord, thank you for lifting off the heavy burden Satan had put on me and putting your gentle yoke upon my shoulders. I can carry your burden because it is gentle and light and a joy to carry. Thank you, Jesus, for saving me from my sinful life and restoring my human dignity. As a person who has been set free, I praise and thank you.

Mustard Seed Faith

And Jesus said unto them, Because of your unbelief: for verily I say unto you, If ye have faith as a grain of mustard seed, ye shall say unto this mountain, Remove hence to yonder place; and it shall remove; and nothing shall be impossible unto you. (Matt. 17:20)

Much too often we limit God by our unbelief and lack of vision. We look at our fat, unhealthy bodies and think, "Well, God can only do so much for me. After all this time, it's almost impossible to help me out completely." This attitude is not uncommon. However, it is only a lack of faith.

The disciples suffered the same problem when they could not expel a demon from a boy and Jesus had to do it for them. When they asked why, Jesus explained that they didn't have enough "living" faith, but with this faith nothing would be impossible to them or us.

When you put that living, active faith (in God) into motion, that fat and flab has to begin melting away; that gluttony has to go; that body of yours has to get in line with what you say. Speak in faith, claim your weight loss and stand on that confession with living faith and you shall surely have what you say.

Lord, sometimes I think, "If only I had the faith of the apostles, then I could really live for God." I realize now, Lord, that I do have "their" faith living in me and that they had problems releasing theirs also. Teach me to activate the faith within me, Lord, and believe you to remove all that fat and wrong eating.

In One Accord

Again I say unto you, That if two of you shall agree on earth as touching any thing that they shall ask, it shall

> be done for them of my Father which is in heaven. For
> where two or three are gathered together in my name,
> there am I in the midst of them. (Matt. 18:19)

Sometimes when a person has climbed on God's bandwagon, he still needs some support from another believer to stand firm. There's power in numbers, but there's even greater power in numbers when the people are praying in one accord for a common goal. Jesus said if two or more agree in faith upon anything (that lines up with the Word, of course) it shall be done. That's exciting!

There's a subtle little word in that Scripture that seems to escape most people but is very significant, and that is the word "for." It means we don't have to do anything but pray in agreement and God will do what we ask—*for* us. That's right, if you've claimed (in faith) victory over compulsive eating, God will do it for you, not expect you to work it out on the basis of your own self-control.

If you haven't prayed the prayer of agreement concerning eating or weight control, do so today. Your husband or wife (if you're married) would be your best partner, but any born-again believer in one accord with God and you will do. Decide on what you wish done, and pray in agreement. Believe you have it, and it shall be yours.

Father, we agree by faith, in Jesus' name, that my weight loss will continue until I am at the weight I should be. We also agree that you will change my eating habits completely and permanently to fit your perfect will. We claim this according to Matthew 18:19, by faith, and believe we have that for which we pray because your Word says so. Thank you now for the results.

Whatever You Ask

> And all things, whatsoever ye shall ask in prayer,
> believing, ye shall receive. (Matt. 21:22)

The apostles saw Jesus perform many miracles, but they never ceased to be amazed by them. In Matthew 21, Jesus had caused a fig tree to wither from its roots, and the apostles were amazed. Jesus told them that with the proper use of their faith, they, too, could do these things and receive whatever they requested.

This promise was not only to the apostles but to all born-again believers. No matter what your dietary need is today, you can claim the answer to that need according to Matthew 21:22. Of course, you must ask according to God's will, but anything asked accordingly can be yours. Do you need to lose ten more pounds? Do you still have trouble resisting forbidden foods at parties? Do commercials still affect you? Whatever your problem, God can and will solve it for you and release you. Stand on His Word, by faith, and hold tight until the answer is manifested. God is faithful to His Word!

Father, you know the needs I have, especially this one. (State your need.) It's so hard to deal with and sometimes I forget you've taken me this far along and that you'll be with me all the way. I claim by faith in Jesus' name that this need will be met, and I thank you in advance for the answer because I receive it right now by faith.

Be on Guard

> Watch and pray, that ye enter not into temptation: the spirit indeed is willing, but the flesh is weak. (Matt. 26:41)

How many times did our spirits and hearts want to quit our gluttonous eating and lose weight in our bodies. Yet, each time we tried, we failed. Each time we thought of dieting, our flesh would react and cry out for a pound of candy or cake or something. Alas, we still have fleshly bodies and they are not oblivious to temptation.

When we turned our eating over to God, He made a great change for the better. He changed our attitudes within and helped quiet our flesh down so that we were able, through Him, to take on a whole new way of eating and living. However, we find out sooner or later that we are not untouched by temptation. At first, God strengthens us and supports us more, but eventually He pulls back so that we will learn to exercise our faith in Him. That's when we really find out that the old flesh is still there.

Jesus warns His disciples not to be closed minded but to pray and be careful that the flesh isn't tempted. Today that is still true for us. We must keep our guard up and avoid temptations as well as exercise faith to combat them when they occur. You can win if you seek God and are aware that temptations will come.

Father, I know my flesh is weak; that's how all this mess started in the first place. Teach me what to look out for that I might avoid giving in to temptation. Thank you, Father, for I know you are watching over me.

Teach Others

And Jesus came and spake unto them, saying, All power is given unto me in heaven and in earth. Go ye therefore, and teach all nations, baptizing them in the name of the Father, and of the Son, and of the Holy Ghost. Teaching them to observe all things whatsoever I have commanded you: and lo, I am with you alway, even unto the end of the world. Amen. (Matt. 28:18-20)

When Jesus died and rose from the dead, He conquered

death, and the dominion which Adam had forfeited to Satan became His. As we accept Jesus and are born into God's family, this dominion becomes ours if we know how to appropriate it. Jesus was telling His disciples that they were to preach and teach to the world those things which they learned from Him, and that He, through the Holy Spirit, would always be with them (and now, us).

Because Jesus regained dominion on earth, we can preach and teach with power those things He teaches us. It is not enough that you realize gluttony really is a sin and that God has set you free, changed your eating habits and helped you lose weight. Now you are called to share this message with others even as it was shared with you.

Seek God on this. Ask Him to show you where, how, and who to witness to. Remember He is with you always, so you're never left alone to tell others. Jesus, through the Holy Spirit, will quicken in you the right words to reach others. Even if it doesn't look like you've broken through to them, keep the faith because God alone knows the results in their hearts.

Father, you've given me so much, but until now I haven't really shared much of it for fear I'd turn someone off. Now I realize it's my duty and privilege to share with others the truths you've shown me. Be with me, Jesus, even as your Word promises you will be, that I might be of help to others.

A Nonverbal Witness

> And John was clothed with camel's hair, and with a girdle of a skin about his loins; and he did eat locusts and wild honey. (Mark 1:6)

John the Baptist was a man set apart from birth for the Lord's service. He was never allowed to drink alcohol nor to shave his head but was holy before God. Since he was set apart for God's work, it is not surprising to see that his diet was different. No alcohol? Locusts and wild honey to eat? Why? Partly to keep him "clean" before God both within and without, he ate God's natural food and abstained from alcohol, which can harm the body and poison the mind if too much is consumed. No, God wanted him clean and above reproach so that when he began preaching the coming of Jesus, people would know that he was legitimately sent of God and following God. One look at him told the whole story.

God hasn't called us to a diet of locusts and honey in the wilderness, but He does expect us to keep our bodies clean and in good shape. He wants people to know just by looking at us that we don't just preach or teach to hear ourselves talking, but that we live each word we say. If our very appearance indicates we live contrary to Jesus' teaching, then our witnessing for Him is hindered or made void. Your appearance isn't only your problem, it's God's. He wants to shape you up and present you to the world as an obviously obedient child.

Are you called of God? Then look and act like it. Get in line with God's will and desire for your eating, and witness nonverbally as well as verbally. See if your results won't be much more dynamic.

Lord, I'm glad that you really understand me and that it is your desire to help me shape up. I know that my outward life must reflect my inward life or people will not take me seriously and I will bring dishonor to you. In Jesus' name, Lord, thank you for your help in this weight battle and for the extra push I needed to keep on keeping on.

Works of Repentance

Bring forth therefore fruits worthy of repentance, and begin not to say within yourselves, We have Abraham to our father; for I say unto you, That God is able of these stones to raise up children unto Abraham. (Luke 3:8)

Good works alone will never get you to heaven; the Word of God makes that clear. However, good works are not obsolete. In fact, for repentance to be valid, we are told there has to be some physical evidence. John the Baptist was telling the people that the fact they were of the seed of Abraham didn't make them exempt from proving their repentance by visible signs.

We can repent all day of the sins of gluttony and poor "temple" care, but as long as we keep shoving in the food by the gallon, particularly junk foods, no one will believe us, especially God. Being a born-again believer doesn't make us exempt. Salvation will get us to heaven, but it won't keep us in God's will. If we do not confess our sins, they will not be forgiven. Realizing you're a glutton and being sorry for it is only half of the requirement; repentance is necessary to remain in fellowship with God.

If you want others (God included) to know that you've repented of gluttony and poor eating habits, then act like it. Don't cheat! "Every once in a while I eat this," could lead to all the time, and where is your fruit of repentance? Remember this the next time you're tempted to eat that pie "just this once": repentance is total!

Lord, I am sorry for being a glutton and compulsive eater all these years. I know my actions must line up with my confession, and they will. Thank you, Lord, in Jesus' name for forgiving me and setting me free to live for you.

The Authority of God's Word

And Jesus being full of the Holy Ghost returned from

Jordan, and was led by the Spirit into the wilderness,
Being forty days tempted of the devil. And in those
days he did eat nothing: and when they were ended
he afterward hungered. (Luke 4:1-2)

Did you ever wonder how Jesus could possibly understand
your temptation by food and know what you were going
through? Have you sometimes doubted that He (or anyone
else, for that matter) did? This Scripture sheds some light on the
subject. We are "starving" if we miss one meal, but Jesus went
forty days and nights without food, and He was *hungry*.

Maybe you've been dieting for a few months and still are very
tempted by some forbidden foods. Every once in a while you
break and you think, "God understands." Well, yes, He does,
but it doesn't have to be that way. You can draw on the same
power and understanding that Jesus did and resist the
temptation.

When Jesus was just coming off the fast, Satan tempted Him
to prove himself by turning the stone into bread. Now you know
that probably sounded really good to Jesus just about then. But
did He do Satan's wishes? He said, "*It is written. . . .*" He used
the power and authority of God's Word to stand in the face of
temptation and not yield to it.

We have the same resources at our command as well as an
understanding "high priest" in Jesus. We can call on the Word
and believe in the power of the blood of Jesus to sustain us
through temptation and bring us out sinless. Jesus understands
your feelings and wants to help you through temptations. Call
on Him when you need to; He's always there.

Father, thank you for sending Jesus to save us and set us free.
I guess I always thought I was alone and fairly helpless when
temptation struck, but I see now that I'm not. I can call on Jesus
and use your Word to resist the temptation. I need never give in
to temptation again.

Captives Set Free

The Spirit of the Lord is upon me, because he hath anointed me to preach the Gospel to the poor; he hath sent me to heal the brokenhearted, to preach deliverance to the captives and recovering of sight to the blind, to set at liberty them that are bruised, To preach the acceptable year of the Lord. (Luke 4:18-19)

When Jesus entered the synagogue in Nazareth on the Sabbath day, He was handed the scroll to read and this was the Scripture He read. When He had finished, He put the scroll down and told the people the Word was fulfilled in Him. Do you know what that means to us? It means Jesus came to save us and meet our every need!

Let's zero in on the last part of the Scripture and see just what it means to the dieter. We certainly have been broken-hearted, but Jesus says one reason He came to us was to heal that broken heart. Next, sight is promised to the blind. Hasn't Jesus given us sight so that we are no longer blind to the evils of gluttony, compulsive eating, and poor nutrition? As we have yielded, He has made our sight of the truth about food clearer and clearer. He has come and given us sight.

Perhaps the most important aspect to the dieter is "deliverance to the captives." How blessed we are that Jesus was sent to set us free—not only from sin but from every bondage that we find ourselves in. He has come to tell us how to be free from gluttony, free from fat, forever.

But the best was saved for last. He came to preach the "acceptable year of the Lord." The Amplified Bible makes that more clear by explaining that this means a time when salvation and free favors profusely abound. We who are born again are living in that "acceptable year," and all of these free favors and salvation are at our fingertips through the power of the blood of Jesus Christ.

Oh, Father, thank you for my freedom, deliverance, and salvation in Christ Jesus. You meet my every need (often before I even ask) and you lift me up when I'm troubled. If I fail to live up to my dietary commitment, you forgive me and set me back on the right path as soon as I come to you with it. Praise you, Father, in Jesus' name.

Cast the Net Once More

And Simon answering said unto him, Master, we have toiled all the night, and have taken nothing: nevertheless at thy word I will let down the net. And when they had this done, they inclosed a great multitude of fishes: and their net brake. (Luke 5:5-6)

If we ever hope to receive from God, we have to have faith in Him and operate without question on His command. When Jesus finished teaching from Peter's boat, He told Peter where to go to catch some fish. Now Peter and his partners had spent the night fishing the area and had caught nothing, but Peter spoke in faith and told Jesus, "On your word I'll do it!" We know from the Scripture that his faith paid off, and the fishermen had so many fish their nets were breaking and they had to call for help to get the fish back to shore.

Jesus doesn't give sparingly; He gives in abundance. We've been out there on the "sea of diets" and tried everything we knew to do in order to lose weight and be free from gluttony and compulsive eating. We really toiled, too, but were out in the night with no luck. Then Jesus told us where to latch on to what we needed to get the results we wanted. Perhaps for some of us it was a diet we'd already tried, but it was our willingness to try one more time for Jesus (on His Word) that brought about abundant results.

Our nets of "dietary knowledge" have been filled to overflowing by Jesus, but what should we do now? We should do what Peter did—call to our friends who need that knowledge and help them to receive the gifts Jesus has given in abundance. Let's not be greedy and keep all these blessings to ourselves; let's share with others every chance we get and give even as we were given to.

Lord, I don't know a lot about fishing, but I know if Peter's nets were breaking they must have been really full. I know that's how my life is with you, in control, and that you've given me so much dietary knowledge and help that I can't help sharing with everyone who desires it. Lord God, your Word satisfies and abounds. I thank and praise you, in Jesus' name.

Fast When Seeking God

> And he said unto them, Can ye make the children of the bridechamber fast, while the bridegroom is with them? But the days will come, when the bridegroom shall be taken away from them, and then shall they fast in those days. (Luke 5:34-35)

"Fast" used to be a dirty word. It meant physical torture. The only reason for doing it was to lose two or three pounds quickly. This is not the Christian attitude concerning fasting, nor should a Christian fast for this reason. The disciples didn't fast as long as Jesus was with them, but did so after He ascended to heaven. Why?

Well, when Jesus was with them, they operated on the power given to them by Him in person. There was no real need to fast as they had Him with them and were celebrating in that respect.

When He left, then they had to exercise faith and seek God through Jesus on a deep spiritual level. In order to get deep into spiritual things, fasting was a tool. It was a part of their normal Christian life just as it can be in yours.

We must get past thinking of fasting in a dietary way and use it as a tool of prayer and seeking God. We, of all people, know it involves sacrifice and discomfort, but we must be willing to give in this way to receive from God. Jesus never said we "could" fast, He said we "would." Make fasting a regular part of your life.

Heavenly Father, for so many years I've thought of fasting as self-torture to remedy last night's eating binge. Forgive me, in Jesus' name, for not seeing my error. Teach me your will concerning fasting in my life and teach me to do so in a proper spirit.

New Wine in New Bottles

But new wine must be put into new bottles; and both are preserved. No man also having drunk old wine straightway desireth new: for he saith, The old is better. (Luke 5:38-39)

Making drastic changes in our lives is never easy. Very rarely do we immediately turn a problem area of our life over to God the minute He begins dealing with us about it. When we were first aware we were guilty of gluttony, poor eating habits, etc., we ignored the truth and kept on trying to work out our "fat" problem on our own. As Jesus said, we weren't really impressed by the seeming strictness of the new life style God was proposing. To us, the old way—like the old wine—looked (tasted) much better.

It's this reality that makes it necessary for God to change us completely within as well as without. If He only changes our outside, our inside attitude would eventually burst through and we'd be fat again. If He only changed the inside, the outside would be no better off and we'd still be fat. In order to really help us, God must bring us to the point of being changed into "new wine" (new dietary life). Our bodies must be "new bottles" (slim bodies) to accept the new way of eating. Only when we yield totally can God change us and make a lasting difference.

It's never easy to make a total dietary change, but it is beneficial when God steps in and makes everything new for us. The process takes time between giving up the old way and really enjoying the taste of the new way, but it's well worth the effort.

Father, thank you for helping me cultivate a taste for the new eating plan you've given me. My taste buds are a little stubborn sometimes and my body isn't excited about this change, but my spirit and heart are soaring for joy!

No Lasting Benefit

> And I will say to my soul, Soul, thou hast much goods laid up for many years: take thine ease, eat, drink, and be merry. But God said unto him, Thou fool, this night thy soul shall be required of thee: then whose shall those things be, which thou hast provided. (Luke 12:19-20)

Our big concern in life was having our kind of food in our kind of quantity (tons preferably). We were willing to let days go by without prayer or feeding on God's Word but wouldn't let hours go by without eating something. This whole earthly society spends its time worrying, working, and getting ulcers all to store up food, clothing, and earthly possessions.

Things were no different in Jesus' day and He called such

worriers fools. What good will a huge house, two cars, a full pantry, and a fat gut do you when it's your time to die? Jesus is saying, why spend your whole life storing up material things (eating, drinking, and getting fat) to please the flesh when they are of no lasting benefit? Rather, work on your relationship with God and grow strong and rich in Him. It's all you'll be "taking with you" when you go.

Of course, food and clothing are important but certainly not worthy of spending a short life on earth to acquire. Like the man in Jesus' parable, people today work with greed as their goal and by the time they have what they want and relax to eat, drink, and be merry, their health is shot, their soul is poor, and their life comes to a tragic end. God has shown us a better way and set us free from this existence.

Lord, I remember what it's like to live to eat and spend money on things that are unimportant in the light of eternal life. I know food and possessions are here for enjoyment, but now I understand that they have a place in life that is low on my priority list. Thank you for re-evaluating my life for me and setting my priorities straight.

Count the Cost

> Or what king, going to make war against another king, sitteth not down first, and consulteth whether he be able with ten thousand to meet him that cometh against him with twenty thousand? (Luke 14:31)

Salvation required a conscious decision on our part. We had to make a choice between going our own way in life and choosing Jesus Christ and His blood sacrifice for our sins. In order to make that choice, we had to consider the consequences of our decision. There's no denying that choosing Jesus involves self-sacrifice, too, and taking up our own cross to die to self. No one chooses salvation without weighing the cost first.

In our daily Christian walk, this same principle comes into play again and again. We are constantly faced with decisions, and if we are wise, we weigh the cost before we make them. The dietary decision is no exception. We have to weigh the cost of yielding our appetite and eating patterns to Jesus and choose Jesus and all He requires of us, or we'll never succeed. Without evaluating the cost, we could very well fail early in the battle by unexpected trials. Wanting to follow Jesus is good, but it isn't enough. You must be willing to die to self in order to live God's way in the area of eating.

Yielding to God means eating only foods He allows, only the quantity He allows, and only for the right reasons. You must face the possibility of physical discomfort for a while and battle against temptation. But, the end result makes it all worthwhile. When the smoke is cleared, you and Jesus will have won the battle.

Lord, I've carefully weighed the cost concerning diet. I know I'll have to give up some foods forever and stop eating as much as I have been. I know it won't be easy sometimes, and I'll wonder why I'm doing it to myself. It's at those times that I ask you to remind me that I'm doing it for you. I want to serve you and be pleasing to you, because you've given me life and happiness and more than I could ever tell. I've counted the cost, decided on you, and am going ahead.

A More Important Food

> But he said unto them, I have meat to eat that ye know not of. (John 4:32).

We like to think of the apostles as being very wise men, but the truth is they were only men who derived their knowledge from Jesus' teaching and the Holy Spirit. When Jesus and His disciples had come into Sychar (in Samaria), the disciples left Jesus near Jacob's well to go buy food. While they were gone, Jesus had the talk with the Samaritan woman and ministered to her. When the disciples returned with food, Jesus told them He had food they didn't know of, and they thought He meant physical food. This shows how earthly-minded they still were.

Today most people think of physical food as the life-sustaining substance. In view of this, don't be surprised if deep concern for you is voiced by family and friends when you start to eat God's way. There will be concern that you aren't eating enough or that you're starving your body and causing yourself physical and emotional pressure. Some may feel you are carrying your religion too far. Whatever the concern, you can answer as Jesus did that your true nourishment is to do God's will in your life. As long as you are in His will and ministering for Him, He will give you all you need for both physical and spiritual strength. You can depend on Him.

It's really exciting, Father, to know I have "food" people don't know about. I know you'll lead me in bodily care, but I realize it is more important that I care for your work both through me and in me. Thank you, Lord, for allowing me to feed on your Word and your work.

Don't Forget the Master

Jesus answered them and said, Verily, verily, I say unto you, Ye seek me, not because ye saw the miracles, but because ye did eat of the loaves, and were filled. Labour not for the meat which perisheth, but for that meat which endureth unto everlasting life, which the Son of man shall give unto you: for him hath

God the Father sealed." (John 6:26-27)

It is recorded several times in the gospels where Jesus multiplied loaves and fishes and fed the crowds because they were hungry after following Him for days. He had compassion on them. But many began to follow Him and hear Him only to receive the food which He gave. They were missing the really important, lasting gift Jesus was offering. Jesus spoke against this and told them not to waste their time on the physical food but to seek after the salvation He offered. The physical food would be gone soon, but the salvation would last.

Unfortunately, many "Christian dieters" today use Jesus the same way. Many see the results in weight loss and eating changes He has brought in other lives, so they jump on the bandwagon and follow Him just to become fat-free and temperate. If this is the extent of your relationship with Jesus, you've missed the boat. The strength and help Jesus gives you in the eating area of your life should be just one of the many results of your following Him and doing His will. Don't try to use Jesus like another fad diet that you idolize today and drop tomorrow. He isn't a tool to use to get slim: He is Lord. Allow Him to help you. Yield to Him your appetite and eating habits, but don't allow this to be your reason for following Him.

Lord, I know that you've helped me so much in weight loss and eating regulation, but please don't let me ever lose sight of the fact that it is you who is important, not what you give. Keep me ever mindful of the important things in life and my motives for following you. Correct me when I start to go wrong and strengthen me in you.

No More Hunger?

And Jesus said unto them, I am the bread of life: he

that cometh to me shall never hunger; and he that believeth on me shall never thirst. (John 6:35)

To say that simply by coming to Him would solve the daily problems of hunger and thirst was boldness on Jesus' part. Many people thought He meant physical food and said, "Yes, give it to us!" But Jesus was talking about something more encompassing than food and drink. He was speaking first of spiritual hunger and thirst and then symbolically speaking of meeting people's basic physical needs as they trusted in Him.

Jesus is in the business of providing. If we have a need or problem, He is there to meet and solve that situation according to God's will, not ours. No more hunger and thirst sounds good. We've spent all of our lives hungry and thirsty for more and more, but Jesus has come to give us satisfaction. As we eat and drink according to God's will, we will be satisfied. This doesn't mean we'll never feel hunger pains or thirst. Unless we eat regularly, we will. It means He'll meet these needs and ease our hunger and thirst. If that's not talking miracles, what is?

Lord, thank you for satisfying the hunger of my soul and spirit and for saving me. Thank you also for teaching me of food and drinks that satisfy and keep me physically strong. Thank you for meeting my total needs through Jesus Christ.

The Spirit is With You

Jesus answered and said unto him, If a man love me, he will keep my words: and my Father will love him, and we will come unto him, and make our abode with him. (John 14:23)

This concept of loving God and showing it by keeping His Word is expressed in John 14, and each time a different "treat" is added by Jesus. Here, Jesus says if we love Him, He and the Father will come to live in us. Of course, we know this is in the form of the Holy Spirit, and we receive Him into our lives at salvation.

Because the Spirit lives in us, He also is always with us, even when we are sinning. Do you realize that the Spirit is right there when you sneak that scoop of ice cream? He's there when you cheat on your diet. He's there day and night. When you open the refrigerator and when you eat that cookie, He is there. How sad He must be at those times; how disappointed He is that we don't reach out to Him for help.

But there's more to it than that. The Spirit is there also when you say no to the ice cream. He's there when you stick to your diet and suffer the pains of temptation. He's there when you open the refrigerator and pick up a carrot instead of a cookie. He's there for all those victories and His joy is sweet because you are showing your love for God!

Which thought is more pleasant and satisfying to you—His joy or sorrow? Which result do you really want to be responsible for? As you face each new situation daily, be conscious of the fact that the Holy Spirit is right there with you. He is there because Jesus and the Father love you and sent Him. With that thought in mind, what could any food really offer that would satisfy?

Father, I've known your Spirit was living in me since I was born again, but sometimes I've forgotten that He is present. I can't hide when I sin, when I cheat on my diet. Your Spirit is there, and I ask you to forgive me, in Jesus' name. I'm glad He's living in me and pray I will bring Him only joy. Remind me of His presence daily, that I might act accordingly and solicit His help when needed.

Be Comforted and Taught

But the Comforter, which is the Holy Ghost, whom the Father will send in my name, he shall teach you all things, and bring all things to your remembrance, whatsoever I have said unto you. (John 14:26)

It was a sad time when Jesus told His disciples He was leaving, but He told them of the promised Comforter (the Holy Spirit) who would be there to teach, comfort, intercede, stand by, and aid. Jesus promised that the Spirit would bring to their remembrance the things He had taught them after He was gone. Of course, we know His Word is true, and the Spirit did come at Pentecost and is here today for those who will allow Him in their lives.

Just as the disciples relied on the teaching of the Spirit to know how to live in God's will, we, too, have this privilege. Books on diet and nutrition are good to read, but we need the teaching of the Holy Spirit. If we are yielded to His teaching and leading, He will lead us into God's perfect will for us. We need never guess in any area of our life nor need we sorrow because the Spirit is here to comfort as well as teach. Not only does the Spirit comfort us in times of dietary temptation, but He uplifts us so that we soar above that temptation in victory as we yield to Him. Let's never be slack in our thanksgiving for the Holy rit, nor underestimate His worth. He is here as our teacher; let Him teach.

Father, thank you for your Holy Spirit. I know He's the best authority on proper nutrition, compulsive eating, etc. Since I'm born again, I'm enrolled in His school. Lord, help me to listen, ask questions, receive answers, and be taught according to your perfect will.

According to His Will

> If ye abide in me, and my words abide in you, ye shall
> ask what ye will, and it shall be done unto you. (John
> 15:7)

The latter part of the verse is exciting and sounds so encompassing, but the first part has to be in practice before the promise can be claimed. We must first live our lives in the will of God as Jesus taught us, as the Word indicates. It is only when we are operating in the perfect will of God that we have such close communion with Him and can boldly ask the desires of our hearts.

"Does this mean I can have anything? Like lots of money, a big car, fame, fortune, a slim body without any dieting, etc?" Well, you tell me. If you are walking in God's perfect will and living by His Word, then you cannot and will not ask anything of Him that is contrary to His teaching. God cannot be manipulated by some secret formula of words you repeat even if they are seemingly scriptural. Unless you use the Word in its proper meaning and context, you will never achieve results.

God will never give you anything He knows is harmful to you or is out of His will for you. However, He will give you anything you ask within His will and according to His Word. You have a right to claim John 15:7 for dietary help, nutrition knowledge, healing of your metabolism, etc. God will grant you a slim, healthy body but on His terms, not yours. In the end, you achieve the desired results and grow in physical and spiritual strength.

Lord, your promises are so precious to me. I know I wouldn't really want you to grant any request of mine that would be contrary to your Word because I know I would regret it later. You know what is good for me, and I trust you to make the right decisions for my life. Thank you, Father, in Jesus' name.

Gluttony Counted as Sin

Who knowing the judgment of God, that they which
commit such things are worthy of death, not only do
the same, but have pleasure in them that do them.
(Rom. 1:32)

This is a very strong Scripture and really hits hard at American
society. In particular, the "things worthy of death" mentioned
included homosexuality, lust, gossiping, jealousy, envy,
gluttony, and greed.

Whether we like it or not, God sees greed and gluttony as sin
worthy of death. The Scripture says God turned such people as
committed these sins over to their own lust and let them reap the
results of their sin. We are fortunate that because of Jesus'
blood, God deals with us less severely. If He gave us what we
deserved, there wouldn't be an overpopulation problem in the
world.

God doesn't require our life of us as in the Old Testament
days, but we do lose a certain part of that life simply because
God allows us to use our free will and suffer the consequences of
our wrong action. Most of us are more than aware of the fact that
greed and gluttony have cost us peace, happiness, good health,
and a good self-image. Gluttony and greed are still sins. God
hasn't forgotten it, and just because "everyone is doing it"
doesn't change one bit of the truth of God's Word. People and
society change, but God's Word remains the same. Sin is sin,
and all sin requires confession and repentance to be washed
away.

Lord, I guess I never really paid much attention to the fact that
gluttony and greed are sins just like idolatry, murder, and
stealing. I confess and repent in Jesus' name and I thank you for
revealing this truth to me.

God is Glorified

And not only so, but we glory in tribulations also: knowing that tribulation worketh patience; and patience, experience; and experience, hope: and hope maketh not ashamed; because the love of God is shed abroad in our hearts by the Holy Ghost which is given unto us. (Rom. 5:3-5)

Diets and changes in eating habits are never easy. When Jesus steps in and heals us and sets us free, this doesn't mean our dieting will be easy sailing. We will have trials, temptations, pressures, and painful hours of waiting. The way we deal with these times and come through them will affect our maturing in Christ. The Word of God says if we want to be victorious and grow in the Spirit, we must be joyful in these times.

In order to be victorious over our trials, we have to transcend them. If we allow them to defeat us by turning around and running, we'll just make it harder on ourselves. We must go through these circumstances, but we should do so joyfully, knowing that we gain patience and steadfastness that matures us in our Christian walk and reinforces our hope of salvation.

Another reason for facing trials joyfully and winning the victory is because in so doing, we stand up for God and don't put Him to shame. He receives the glory due Him, and we show forth His Holy Spirit living in us. So you see, there's more than yourself to think about when that diet gets to be almost too much and you're thinking of breaking it. It's God's business because His witness as well as your spiritual growth is at stake. In light of that fact, how much do you really need that piece of candy? Is that pressure really too hard to resist in joy knowing that you'll grow and glorify the Father?

Father, I guess it's a hard thing to ask me to suffer trials and temptations and be joyful about it. But I really believe I can do it for you. I've always wished I were a patient person. Now I know I can be, but the hard way is the only way to make it. When I consider all Jesus suffered in joy knowing all the good that would come of His pain, I know I can suffer the discomfort of diet and change in my eating habits because good will come of it. Thank you, Father, that I know the joy is there.

New Life in Him

Let not sin therefore reign in your mortal body, that ye should obey it in the lusts thereof. Neither yield ye your members as instruments of unrighteousness unto sin: but yield yourselves unto God, as those that are alive from the dead, and your members as instruments of righteousness unto God. (Rom. 6:12-13)

When we were born again into God's kingdom, we were given life where before we were dead of sin. Many of us accepted that new life in our hearts and souls but have not brought our bodies in line. The Word says that our flesh, too, should be reborn in that we should no longer sin by using our bodies for unrighteousness. As long as our bodies control us and we give in to their desires, we are not totally yielded to God and have not allowed Him to change us totally and give us the new life He wants us to have. We've known this but haven't applied it to the subject of weight loss and eating habits. The devil has kept us thinking it was just "our problem" and there was nothing religious about it. Everything we do is spiritual in nature, either for the good or for the bad.

Now that the Lord has shown us this, He has also given us an alternative way to live and an alternative use of our bodies. Yielding our appetite and lusts to God is not just a giving-up (passive) move, but a gaining (active) move. We are then free to work with all that we have to promote the gospel in every area of our lives. Hallelujah!

Lord, thank you for setting me free. I knew I had to give up the old ways of eating and the sins they lead to, but now I'm really excited because the new way you've given me is a productive tool for witness and righteousness. I know each day when I rise and notice my body slimming, and choose to eat moderately from your good food, that I am not only helping myself, but I am pleasing you and working for you. Father, I just thank and praise you, in Jesus' name, for that privilege.

Power of Sin is Broken

For the law of the Spirit of life in Christ Jesus hath made me free from the law of sin and death. For what the law could not do, in that it was weak through the flesh, God sending his own Son in the likeness of sinful flesh, and for sin, condemned sin in the flesh. (Rom. 8:2-3)

Thank God that Jesus set us free from the law of sin and death and put us under His grace instead. The law was not strong because the fleshly lust of man weakened it. But Jesus came and became an offering for sin. He fought the fleshly battles, won, and broke sin's power. This same power can be ours today; we can do even as Jesus did through the power of the Holy Ghost.

Diverse diets are like the law; they are only as good as the willingness of the flesh to submit. Since the flesh wills to have its own lust and desires, it is not willing to submit for long. Consequently, most diets fail. But when we yield to the Spirit, we gain the victory over that law. We no longer operate by fleshly weakness but draw on the power of God to win the victory.

If you've been trying to practice the principles of Christian weight control without tapping into the source of power, you won't make it. As long as fleshly weakness has room to sneak in, failure is inevitable. Only when we rely totally on the Lord to free us and sustain us can we achieve victory over our eating and achieve lasting results.

Father, I realize even a good plan can't work without the power and authority to put it into action. Thank you, Jesus, for coming to set us free and for winning the victory over fleshly sin so that we might taste of that victory, too. I know I have your plan and your power and authority to make it work.

For Our Good

> And we know that all things work together for good to them that love God, to them who are the called according to his purpose. (Rom. 8:28)

Nothing ever happens in our lives that God doesn't know about. God is aware of our fat, gluttony, compulsive eating and greed and our need for help, even before we ask for that help. He does not want to see us going on and on in our lust for food only to grow fatter and more miserable than ever, but we don't listen to Him or allow Him to help us.

When we cry out for help, the Lord is there and He comes to our rescue. Now we know that we didn't become a fat glutton overnight so we shouldn't expect to become slim and temperate overnight either. The way the Lord has shown us to go is at times painful, but once we've yielded to God, the Word says *all* things work for our good. He has called us to get our appetite under control, and because we love Him, we will do it. At times we wonder about some of the tests and ordeals we go through, but we can stand firm on the Word and know that whatever happens will be for our good.

Father, I don't always understand the things that happen to me, but I know your Word is true. Sometimes it seems I can't turn around without temptation or criticism staring me in the face. I don't know the reason for it all, but I rest in the fact that as I follow your purpose for me it will all work to my good. I just thank and praise you, in Jesus' name.

Nothing Can Separate Us

> For I am persuaded, that neither death, nor life, nor angels, nor principalities, nor powers, nor things present, nor things to come, nor height, nor depth, nor any other creature, shall be able to separate us from the love of God, which is in Christ Jesus our Lord. (Rom. 8:38-39)

Nothing feels more lonely than the feeling of separation from God for a Christian. Satan tries his best to encourage such feelings, but God's Word says it doesn't have to be that way. Even when our sin causes a break in communications with God, the Word says nothing can keep God's love from flowing to us, thanks to Jesus.

For the dieter, one of the worst feelings of separation comes when we've blown it and cheated on our diets. We feel as if we'll never be able to face God again with our failures. The Word says that kind of thinking is wrong. When we love the Lord and come to Him confessing our sins and yielding to His will, *nothing* can keep us separated. What we've done in the past can't because it has been forgiven. Satan can't because we have the victory over him through the blood of Jesus. Friends can't keep us from Him, nor can any who count themselves our enemies. Through His death and resurrection, Jesus has opened communications between us and God forever.

Don't let one failure keep you thinking God has washed His hands of you. Don't go deeper into sin and disobedience because the devil is trying to make you believe it doesn't matter now. Confess, repent, and feel God's love. He cares for you and wants to communicate with you. Don't shut Him out. Claim the privilege of experiencing His love, not allowing anyone or anything to stand in the way.

Father, sometimes I'm so disgusted with myself for failing you, and I let the devil convince me I was shut from you and your love. Thank you, Lord, for showing me he's a liar and that there isn't a separation between us. Lord, I claim that promise that nothing can separate us, and I thank and praise you for it.

Be an Overcomer

Be not overcome of evil, but overcome evil with good. (Rom. 12:21)

God would never tell us to do something we weren't capable of. Therefore, if He tells us to overcome evil with good, we know for certain that we can do just that. Putting this principle into effect concerning diet, we can say that we can overcome gluttony with temperance and fatness with weight loss. Not only can we do these things, but the Word says we're supposed to. We're not to let things like gluttony, greed, compulsive eating, and fatness overcome us.

If we continue to eat temperately, the lust of gluttony has no opportunity to flair up. If we continue to diet faithfully as God has shown us, fat has no way of remaining. We can control our bodies through the power God has given us.

Therefore, it is up to us to replace the sin, replace evil with the good and thereby cancel the evil out. When we only allow good and right thinking and acting in our bodies, only good results can thrive. The choice is ours.

Father, thank you for making it possible for me to live in victory. I'm glad that I can overcome evil with good. I just praise you for providing a way for me to do what is good and right in order that evil might not have a hold in my life.

Anything is Edible?

> For the kingdom of God is not meat and drink; but righteousness, and peace, and joy in the Holy Ghost. (Rom. 14:17)

We've heard this Scripture used a hundred times to prove a hundred different viewpoints, but let us look at it in the context of which it was written. Chapter fourteen talks about not judging people because of what they do or don't eat. Paul is discussing those who would and wouldn't eat meat offered to idols because of their beliefs.

If you wish to twist this Scripture, you can say God says *anything* is acceptable for anyone to eat. This is not so; if we eat anything in ignorance that is bad for us, it is not sin. But to willfully eat something we know is harmful to us or that God has asked us to give up is sin.

Verse fourteen states that the kingdom of God isn't getting food and drink that we *desire,* but it is the joy and peace we receive standing righteous before God. God has put eating and drinking restrictions on each individual for a purpose. Listen to God and learn of His limitations for you. Remember, if you begin to feel rebellious about giving up a food that is proven harmful, it's probably because that food controls you. If you can't seem to give it up, don't try to justify yourself by saying you haven't been convicted. Face the truth and let God deliver you. Stand righteous before Him.

Father, help me never to be critical of others. Teach me to pray for their needs. I haven't been willing to give up some things because it was too hard on me, but I see that's only because they have too much of a hold in my life. Set me free in Jesus' name. I yield it all to you and thank you.

A Temple of God

Know ye not that ye are the temple of God, and that the Spirit of God dwelleth in you? (1 Cor. 3:16)

If studied in its totality, this verse is speaking of the church as a body as well as an individual body in which His Spirit dwells. We, as dieters, are concerned with both aspects. The church as a body needs to keep itself free and clean from sin and false teaching. This includes teaching on the subject of food, weight control, and eating habits. A church body that condones gluttony, greed, and poor eating habits is corrupting God's temple as is the individual Christian who harbors such unscriptural beliefs.

The Word says that anyone who corrupts and defiles God's holy temple will also be corrupted with death for it. If we truly believe we have the Spirit of God within us, how can we keep damaging that "temple" selfishly? Remember, your body is the temple of the Holy Spirit; keep it clean for Him and for yourself.

Lord, keep me ever mindful that my body is the temple in which your Spirit dwells. I want it to be a holy, liveable place for Him to be. Remind me, Lord, when I am not giving that temple proper care, that I might seek forgiveness and be cleansed and made holy again.

Discipline Your Body

And every man that striveth for the mastery is temperate in all things. Now they do it to obtain a corruptible crown; but we an incorruptible. I therefore so run, not as uncertainly; so fight I, not as one that beateth the air: But I keep under my body, and bring it into subjection: lest that by any means, when I have preached to others, I myself should be a castaway. (1 Cor. 9:25-27)

Paul certainly does lay it on the line for us in these few verses. He tells us that we have to control our bodies at all times. Like athletes in training, we need to keep temperate and build our bodies and spirits strong for an eternal crown, not just one moment of earthly glory.

We don't diet, lose weight, and firm our bodies just so we can look nice and get compliments. This will be a result of our efforts but not the main reason for them. Our first reason has to be keeping our bodies under subjection that we might live the temperate, Christ-like life we are called to live. It is not a six-months-a-year thing; it is a life-long practice. We must continue to train, build up, and discipline our bodies, so that we continue to live and walk in the Spirit, not the flesh.

Paul says it won't do us any good to have preached to others God's total gospel if we fail to live it and come out lacking in the end ourselves. We must go forward. We must discipline our bodies each day so that we control them and they never control us again. This is the walk of victory in Christian weight control and "temple" maintenance.

Father, keep me ever mindful that I must stay on top of my

body, disciplining it and strengthening it, never allowing it to control me. You know that I want the temperance I've never had before, Lord. Teach me daily to grow strong in body and spirit.

A Way of Escape

> There hath no temptation taken you but such as is common to man: but God is faithful, who will not suffer you to be tempted above that ye are able; but will with the temptation also make a way to escape, that ye may be able to bear it. (1 Cor. 10:13)

To some of us, this Scripture brings bad and good news. The good news is that no temptation comes along that is not able to be withstood or handled by us, and that God is faithful not to give us more than we can handle. Now to some, the bad part is when God makes us able to bear the temptation.

God has never promised we'd breeze by on this diet, never having to face tests that try us. In fact, He says we'll go through these tests, but we have His Word that He'll never allow a test that we aren't able to handle and pass if we trust in Him. As we turn to Him, He will show us the way through and give us the strength to make it. This may not sound like much fun to some, but it really is exciting to know that we can come through any temptation that comes along. We have God's word on it.

Jesus was tempted in every way we are, but He didn't sin. He chose God's way through each trial that He might show us the way and win the victory as an example to us. We are to use the same tactics Jesus used when temptation comes and that is the sword of God's Word. It works every time we apply Therefore, use it!

Father, I'm excited because your Word assures me I can be

the winner over temptation every time it comes against me if I will turn to you and use your Word as a weapon against the devil. Father, just knowing I don't have to give in to temptation, I am encouraged as I diet and change my eating habits.

All Things New

Therefore if any man be in Christ, he is a new creature: old things are passed away; behold, all things are become new. (2 Cor. 5:17)

We have spent years feeling depressed, frustrated and unhappy about our lives because inside we knew what we were. Now that the Lord has shown us the way out and set us free, we must learn to accept the fact that we are not the way we used to be and we need to learn to see ourselves in a new light. When we got saved, we didn't look too different on the outside, but the Word says we became totally new creatures inside, where it really counts.

This truth manifests itself each time we grow in a certain area of our spiritual walk and yield to God. He makes us new or renewed in that area. The day we yielded all that fat, gluttony, greed, compulsive eating, etc., to God, we didn't immediately become slim and trim, eating tiny portions of food with no problem. We were changed from within, and the outward manifestation is still in the process of being worked out.

If we are to see ourselves as temperate, healthy eaters, we have to recognize that the change begins within us. We are different despite all the fat and flab. We were made new and daily we progress toward the time we will show outwardly that inward change. Don't believe the devil's lie. You are changed, free in Christ.

Lord, please help me to see the inside me that you see.

Sometimes when I look in the mirror I have a hard time believing I'm any different from what I used to be. I know you've changed me within, Lord; just quicken that in my heart.

Your Weakness is an Asset

And he said unto me, My grace is sufficient for thee: for my strength is made perfect in weakness. Most gladly therefore will I rather glory in my infirmities, that the power of Christ may rest upon me. (2 Cor. 12:9)

We are usually not willing to face trials and attacks from the devil without wanting God to get us out of it right away. When we first begin dieting, every temptation we face seems to be too much and we're sure we'll fail. It's at those times God lets us know that we sometimes have to face trials, and when we do, that His grace will pull us through.

One of the most exciting realizations in this Scripture is that our weakness is an asset. Can you believe that? When we are weak, God can use us because we know we can't do anything ourselves. We know it is He who wins the battle. If He doesn't do it for us, we can't make it. God's strength shows through when we are weak because it is obvious to us and those around us that supernatural intervention is taking place.

As an example of God's strength showing through, remember all the diets you've been on, all the times you've tried to be temperate but just couldn't make it. You were weak-willed and went right back on a binge. But when you yielded that area of your life to God, He was able to step in and sustain you through the trials. It was easier for you to yield to God because you were sure you couldn't do it yourself. After all, you'd spent years trying to do it your way with no success. So then it is our

129

weakness and recognition of it that makes us usable to God and gives us a chance to show God's strength to the world.

Lord, I've always been so unhappy because my will is so weak, but now I see that sometimes it can be an asset to me if I yield it to you to be used by you. When you work miracles in me, the world can really see your strength because of my obvious weakness.

No Extra Burdens

> Stand fast therefore in the liberty wherewith Christ hath made us free and be not entangled again with the yoke of bondage. (Gal. 5:1)

No one is so sure of himself that he doesn't need some uplifting once in a while. We should both give and receive uplifting words to keep us strong in the faith. God set us free from the bondage of fat and gluttony, but it's up to us to walk in that freedom. When Jesus saved us, He freed us from sin, death, and bondage of the flesh, but we are not to use that freedom for our own selfish purposes.

There's a two-fold message for the dieter in this Scripture. First, it is an assurance that God has set us free from the world and that we should not allow the devil to put that yoke of bondage on us again. Second, we need to realize that just because we are free from gluttony and greed, we cannot eat as we please. We must keep on top of things using our freedom to enjoy food but our wisdom to weed out some foods and abstain from others.

The Scripture talks about circumcision, and that it was not necessary to put that extra burden on the Gentile converts. Let us also be mindful not to put a whole lot of unnecessary rules and regulations on those who have just been set free from compulsive eating. Let the Lord show them in His perfect time what He would have them to do. Be uplifting that we all may enjoy our liberty.

Father, keep me ever mindful of the freedom you've given me that I might not allow anyone to take it from me. But just as importantly, keep me from robbing my brothers and sisters of their newly acquired liberty also. Teach us all to be supportive of each other and grow in your freedom.

Temperance is a Fruit

> But the fruit of the Spirit is love, joy, peace, longsuffering, gentleness, goodness, faith, meekness, temperance; against such there is no law. (Gal. 5:22-23)

Did you know that "temperance" is a "fruit"? That's right, temperance is a fruit of the Spirit and what are we supposed to do with the fruits of the Spirit? The same thing an apple tree does with apples—produce them.

As with any fruit of the Spirit, temperance must be nurtured by the Word before it will produce a good, ripe fruit. As we produce some of the other fruit (such as faith, longsuffering, etc.) we also produce the basics necessary for temperance to thrive.

With each day of compulsive eating, we stifled the growth of that fruit. The longer we were gluttons, the further we got from producing temperance. Now that we know better, let's strive to produce the good fruit of temperance because the more we produce, the further away we get from the fruitless, miserable days.

Lord, I want to bear the good fruit of temperance one hundred-fold. I spent so many years producing the effects of harmful gluttony, but now that's all over and I want the sweet fruit of temperance. Thank you for showing me this is a fruit of the Spirit, and that because the Spirit lives in me, I should be manifesting that fruit.

Sow Profitably

Be not deceived; God is not mocked: for whatsoever a man soweth, that shall he also reap. For he that soweth to his flesh shall of the flesh reap corruption; but he that soweth to the Spirit shall of the Spirit reap life everlasting. (Gal. 6:7-8)

As sowers to the flesh we certainly wanted to avoid talking about the sowing and reaping principle. We tried to apply it only to sin and stay away from its obvious spiritual and physical application to our lives. In our hearts, we knew every time we sowed three thousand extra calories, we reaped on extra pound of fat on our bodies. What we really didn't want to think about was the other damage to our internal organs that couldn't be as readily seen but was there just the same.

The Word clearly says if your works (like eating) are fleshly and lustful (like gluttony and compulsive eating) then your bodies will reap the effects of decay, ruin, and death. Those are the facts. God said it, and it can't be gotten around.

"But, I've repented of my sin of gluttony, changed my eating, and I still have some physical problems like fat. Why?" Well, God promised to forgive and He did, but you are still reaping what you've sown in the past. It will take a lot of time sowing good food and good eating habits to reap weight loss and health. This is all the more reason not to delay a day longer. Haven't you been reaping the devil's trash long enough? Start sowing good food, good diet, good nutrition, and temperance, and start reaping weight loss, health, controlled appetite.

Father, I've spent too many years sowing gluttony and reaping fat. I've always realized in the back of my mind that I was reaping what I had sown, but I just ignored it. Thank you for making it clear for me and giving me your assurance that as I sow good eating habits and good nutrition, I'll reap a slim, healthy body.

It is by Grace Only

For by grace are ye saved through faith; and that not of yourselves: it is the gift of God: Not of works, lest any man should boast. (Eph. 2:8-9)

The people of Ephesus are reminded here by Paul that their salvation is a free gift from God, and that it cannot be earned. God's salvation is always that way. When He saves us from temptation or a particular sin, it is strictly by our yielding to His grace, for we have no ability to save ourselves.

So often we get to depending on a certain diet or our own determination, and we feel like we're working out our weight loss program. Let's not fall into that trap. It is God's grace that sustains us and brings results. We have no right to become puffed up and egotistical about how well we're doing.

Without faith in God, we would still be wallowing in the pigpen of gluttony, just as without faith in God for our eternal life, we'd still be wallowing in worldly sin and eternal damnation. It is our faith in God's faithfulness to save us that brings us salvation. Let's be ever mindful of the fact that we cannot be free from gluttony, except by God's grace. It is He who deserves the honor and glory!

Father, I give you all the praise and honor and glory. There's nothing I can do to save myself, no matter how hard I might try.

But you are able to give me liberty by your grace. Thank you for the weight loss, change in eating, change in my spiritual life.

Equipped for Battle

Put on the whole armour of God, that ye may be able
to stand against the wiles of the devil. (Eph. 6:11)

This battle of weight loss and eating patterns hasn't really been a matter of us versus food; it is much deeper than that. We've been fighting with "powers and principalities," and it's no wonder we've been defeated for so long; we didn't even know our enemy. There's no way we could have won because we were fighting with all the wrong weapons. We hurled darts of "will power" and "self-discipline" at that food, and it had little effect. The Word tells us we're to use the whole armour of God.

"But what is that? How do I use it?" First, realize that it's a spiritual battle. We fight this battle just as Jesus himself did after forty days and nights in the desert. We put on truth (God's truth and righteousness) as our clothing. We put on our shoes of the gospel of peace. We hold up faith as a shield against the enemy's attacks, and charge ahead with the sword, God's Word. The covering for our heads should be salvation because without it, the battle is already lost. When we are prepared and equipped in this way, we will win the weight loss battle, the eating battle, and any other battle the enemy cares to wage.

Until we understand it isn't the food itself that is causing the problem but rather the forces of the devil trying to control our lives, we cannot hope to achieve lasting results. We must know our enemy and never fear him because we have the more powerful weapons. The victory is already ours through Christ Jesus.

Lord, it's so easy to think food is the problem in itself, but I recognize now that food is only an instrument used by the devil to try to keep me in bondage. Thank you for making clear the battle plan and equipping me with the necessary weapons for a sure victory.

Completing the Work

Being confident of this very thing, that he which hath begun a good work in you will perform it until the day of Jesus Christ. (Phil. 1:6)

Isn't it exciting to know that God isn't through with us yet? We're losing weight, eating better, and growing in temperance, but we know we have a long way to go. We've lived so much of our life the wrong way and now we have a whole new way of life to look forward to. But we know it will be an ongoing work the rest of our lives.

Too many times we want to jump the gun on God. He gives us a little bit of wisdom and knowledge on a subject (like Christian weight control) and soon we begin thinking we really know a lot. We decide we really "have it" now, and we charge ahead on our own, not seeking God's will and guidance any longer. Because we have some basic truths, we think we can take it from there and do it all by ourselves. Of course, past experiences have shown that when we do this, we fail terribly.

God never promised to tell it all to us, then let us take it from there. No, He said He'd continue the good work He started in us and do so until we go to be with Him. Remember, we don't know it all, so let's let God lead, and never fail to seek His advice and guidance. Therein lies the true victory in Jesus.

Father, forgive me for thinking I can do it all without you. Keep teaching me and guiding me. Continue to work in my life until I go to be with you. I thank and praise you, in Jesus' name.

Rejoice Always

Rejoice in the Lord alway: and again I say, Rejoice.
Let your moderation be known unto all men. The
Lord is at hand. (Phil. 4:4-5)

When we're losing weight easily, temptation seems like a
thing of the past. Friends and family are being supportive, and
we're looking and feeling good. It's really easy to rejoice and be
glad. But the Word says, *always*! Well now, does that really
mean at all times? Yes, it does!

We face times of stress when trials come upon us, and our first
instinct is to blow up, fall apart or be depressed, but the Word
says we must rejoice because it will all be a good experience in
some way. If it seems we're not losing any weight, and
everywhere we turn there's almost unbearable temptation, we
are still to rejoice because we're learning patience and building
our spiritual strength.

If we are walking in God's will, nothing will befall us that will
be really harmful or damaging. The Lord knows what He is
doing, and if everything is closing in around us and we feel we'll
explode at any minute, we need to get happy because we're in
line for a miracle from God.

The Scripture also says we should let our moderation be
known: Let others see it. Confess it before others. The reason is:
The Lord is at hand. We ought to be living sober, temperate
lives, rejoicing in all things because He is on His way. Even the
problems of this world will mean nothing when He arrives for us.
Let's rejoice today for the King is coming.

Father, when I remember that Jesus is coming for me soon, I
get happy. When things seem to be going wrong, remind me
that you have everything under control and that there's a good
reason for what's happening. Teach me to rejoice when it's easy

and when it's not so easy.

Worry About Nothing

Be careful for nothing; but in everything by prayer and supplication with thanksgiving let your requests be made known unto God. And the peace of God, which passeth all understanding, shall keep your hearts and minds through Christ Jesus. (Phil. 4:6-7)

Can you imagine in this world of turmoil and confusion, God asking and expecting us not to be anxious or worried about anything? He does, and we know He never asks us to do anything we are not able to. As compulsive eaters we had all kinds of fears and anxieties. We worried about being rejected because we were fat. We were anxious every time we had to lose weight for some occasion. Before one meal was finished we were already worried about the next one as if we'd starve to death between the two. Needless to say, we certainly weren't trusting God.

Now that we are walking in God's will and He is in control, we are not to worry. The Word says to go before Him in prayer and inquire about our needs and thank Him in advance. We no longer worry about weight loss; we've asked and He is working it out. He is teaching us temperance, meeting our every need. Instead of worrying, we can rest assured that God is taking care of everything and His peace can fill the area where anxiety once existed.

The Word says our minds and hearts will be at complete peace if we go to God when problems arise, turn them over to Him, and really believe He'll take care of them. Then we thank Him and are at peace in Him. As we trust God, He gives inner peace, deeper than man can comprehend.

Father, I always thought worrying was just a part of life we had to live with, but I realize now that if I'm trusting you completely, there's never a need to worry about anything. I wish to experience your perfect peace in my walk with you. Thank you for your provision.

Guard Your Thoughts

> Finally, brethren, whatsoever things are true, whatsoever things are honest, whatsoever things are just, whatsoever things are pure, whatsoever things are lovely, whatsoever things are of good report; if there be any virtue, and if there be any praise, think on these things. (Phil. 4:8)

One of a compulsive eater's biggest enemies is his mind. Our minds can really get us into trouble. We start to think about a certain food and instead of doing something else to resist that food, we begin to dwell on that thought. Now, you say to yourself, "We all know thinking about eating isn't wrong." Well, it certainly is, and the more we think about it, the more likely we are to break down and have an eating binge. We have to learn to control our thoughts. Granted, wrong thoughts will enter our minds, but it's up to us how far they go. We can reject the thoughts immediately and avoid a difficult struggle or we can entertain the thought, struggle, and end up eating what we shouldn't.

We need to learn how to test each thought that comes into our minds and reject those that are improper. For this reason, the Scripture was given that we might have some guidelines for testing our thoughts. We are to think on the good things—things that are good for us, not the "goodies" that got us in such sad shape. If as dieters we fix our minds on temperance and do not dwell on thoughts of food, we will find ourselves more than able to deal with temptations when they come.

Father, teach me to resist wrong thoughts as soon as they come to my mind. I am in control, and through you I know I can choose what I think. As I renew my mind, help me to fill it with pleasant, uplifting thoughts and thereby make my life happier, easier, and more directly in your will.

Whether Full or Hungry

I know both how to be abased, and I know how to abound: everywhere and in all things I am instructed both to be full and to be hungry, both to abound and to suffer need. I can do all things through Christ which strengtheneth me. (Phil. 4:12-13)

To be out of food, even for a short time, used to be the biggest disaster we could encounter. Now that Jesus is the leader, we need to reevaluate our feelings. We must realize that there's nothing we cannot endure if Christ is our strength. We can bear hunger, and we can enjoy food without overdoing it. We are no longer slaves to our appetites.

Paul says he's been hungry and full, and both are the same because Jesus is the true, constant need in his life. As long as that need is met, all others are met in one way or another. We, too, have to accept Jesus as our one important need in life, and when we do, we can rest, knowing our needs are met in Him.

Abundance and lack are equally good for us. If we lack, we learn to depend more heavily on God and grow closer to Him. Also, we learn to appreciate more fully what we do have. When there's abundance, we rejoice and are filled with happiness, and that, too, is good for us. From time to time on our diets, God will cause us to lack some food we enjoy, but it is only for our teaching and strengthening. We must learn that earthly things are not of prime importance in our life because they will one day be done away with. It is our spiritual needs that are most important. When we learn to do without and be content, it is then that God can give us abundantly, knowing it will not harm our growth.

Father, after all these years of loving and craving food, I really do need to learn to "take it or leave it." It's a hard lesson for me, but a good one, so teach me as you see fit. I want to be able to say I'm happy and resting in you no matter how much or how little food I have. Thank you, Lord, for the life-changing lesson I know you are willing to give me.

Vain Philosophy

Beware lest any man spoil you through philosophy and vain deceit, after the tradition of men, after the rudiments of the world and not after Christ. For in Him dwelleth all the fulness of the Godhead bodily. And ye are complete in him, which is the head of all principality and power. (Col. 2:8-10)

This Scripture cautions us to be very careful not to fall into the trap of man's philosophy and put ourselves into bondage. We are to function on a spiritual plane. Unless we do, we can very easily fall victim to the foolishness of this world. We are to take care not to be involved with those who seek to explain all problems and situations away by psychology and intellectualism.

There are many books today on diet that state that the problems are psychological, and proceed to offer solutions accordingly. These methods never reach down to the root problem of sin and disobedience to God. Then there is the modern school of thought which basically claims to "affirm" and "support" the compulsive eater, by trying to convince him that he's really "okay" and that he should love himself (and others should love him) just the way he is. This teaching says there's no need for weight or dietary change because the person is beautiful as he is and should be content with himself. This philosophy is contrary to the teachings of Jesus and God's Word. It encourages the sins of gluttony, greed, vanity, pride, and idolatry.

We are to avoid this way of thinking. If we are to remain in God's will as Christians, we must face our sin and know that we are nothing without Him. Unless we are willing to give up our sins of gluttony and greed, He cannot and will not help us. Unless we are spiritually minded in all things, we cannot walk in victory. We are called to separate ourselves from worldliness and to guard against vain philosophy. Unless we avoid them, we will once more be in bondage.

Lord, the world is full of people saying the mind is the answer to everything, but I know my mind is just a creation of yours. Help me to avoid those who would try to use psychology and vain deceit to put me into bondage. I am free in you and wish to operate my life by faith in you. Thank you, Lord, for warning me of the problems of worldliness.

Meditate on the Word

Let the Word of Christ dwell in you richly in all wisdom; teaching and admonishing one another in psalms and hymns and spiritual songs, singing with grace in your hearts to the Lord. (Col. 3:16)

Have we, as Christians, been living up to the words of this Scripture? Have the words which Jesus spoke been living in their fullness in our hearts so that we live by them and share them with others? Do we go before the Lord singing hymns and psalms as a joyful worship to Him? If the answer is no, we need to make some changes.

Before we can share the Word with each other, teaching, admonishing, and uplifting one another, we first have to get it into our own hearts. We spend so much time on physical food, planning, preparing, and eating to have strong and healthy bodies; but we also need to spend plenty of time on spiritual food (the Word) to grow strong in the Spirit. We need to set aside times of the day, just as with physical food, to read and share the Word. In order to feast, we must recognize our spiritual hunger and feed it God's Word.

Once we are equipped, we can then share with others. If we have the Word in our hearts concerning food and diet, we can share that and teach others of the deliverance and peace that can be theirs. It is our duty and privilege to share with others. Also, as we keep our minds stayed on sharing and worshiping God, we are less apt to head for the refrigerator out of idleness. We will be snacking instead on God's Word and His truth, building our spirits up, not tearing our bodies down.

Lord, your Word is so precious to me. Since I discovered the wealth of happiness and peace that it brings, I have grown to appreciate it more and more. Help me to share what I've learned with others that they might be uplifted and taught also. Remind me when I'm down to sing songs and hymns of praise to you and uplift my spirit. I adore you and give you all thanks and praise.

All in Jesus' Name

And whatsoever ye do in word or deed, do it all in the name of the Lord Jesus, giving thanks to God and the Father by him. (Col. 3:17)

Can we honestly say that everything we do, we do in the name of Jesus and with dependence on Him? Jesus certainly doesn't approve of gluttony and would never be supportive of such an act. When we fantasize all day about gooey desserts and lust for large amounts of food, can we really claim our thoughts are lined up with Jesus' Spirit? Of course not. We cannot present such thoughts as unto the Lord.

Before we can meet the requirements of Colossians 3:17, we must first get our thoughts and actions in line with God's Word. We must be aware of the things we say and do that we might know what has to be removed from our lives. Any thought or action that is not in line with the Word of God certainly cannot be done as unto God.

It is clear also that we are not to live this way grudgingly or unwillingly. We are to do so in thanksgiving to the Father. It is good to be free to think and act as unto the Lord with His guidance instead of bondage to food and lust. That we might grow more perfect in Him, let us line up our thoughts and actions with the Word and present ourselves before Him in all things.

Lord, I never really thought about presenting everything I say and do before you, as if I were doing it unto you. That certainly makes me more conscious of the things I say and do. Remind me when I stray in thought or action that I might repent and correct that area.

Constant Hotline

Pray without ceasing. In everything give thanks: for this is the will of God in Christ Jesus concerning you. (1 Thess. 5:17-18)

One of the aspects of Christian life is knowing the will of God.

It is usually treated as a very deep, awesome thing, but the truth is God is quite clear about His will when we get into His Word. One aspect of His will is that we be continually in prayer. "But how can I do that?" It is easy to continue in prayer because prayer is speaking or communicating with God, keeping in touch. We should be in constant touch with God. As dieters this is especially important. Unless we are talking with and listening to God constantly, we find we fail in the battle over temptation. If we are in prayer always, wrong thoughts cannot take hold and drag us down into the bakery, refrigerator, pantry, etc.

Another area of God's will is to give thanks in everything. "You mean I should thank God even though I haven't lost any weight in two weeks?" That's what the Word says. God knows what He is doing and has a good reason for everything, but we must trust Him to work it all out. It is not a good characteristic for a Christian to complain and gripe. We are to be governed by love and trust in God. If we are, then we can thank Him in all things knowing that good will come out of all He does.

Father, no wonder I've had such a hard time reaching you sometimes; I had to stop and dial your number when I should have had you on the line all the time. Thank you for showing me that my daily walk includes constant communication with you. I'm glad you reminded me to be thankful in all things because if I trust you, there's no need to complain. Lord, I get so excited as I learn more of you and I just praise you for your love and patient teaching.

Deliverance is Free

Not by works of righteousness which we have done, but according to his mercy he saved us, by the washing of regeneration and renewing of the Holy Ghost. (Titus 3:5)

One of the traps the dieter falls into is the "do-it-yourself" trap. Success or failure is strictly up to you, and usually failure is inevitable. Thank God, that we as Christians have found a better way of weight control through the power of the Holy Spirit.

Just as salvation is free and there is nothing we can do to earn it, so is any gift of God. There are qualifications we must meet, but in no way can we earn the gift by our own goodness. In the case of weight control and eating habits, we know that no amount of good intentions or self-discipline ever really helped; we were still miserable gluttons. But when God stepped in, He worked a miracle in us because of His mercy, not our good works. If we are to continue in success, we must be ever reminded that God is the power behind our victory, not us. Should we fail to remember and try to "work it out from here on our own," we will soon be back to our old way of life and wondering where we went wrong.

God's mercy is what brings results—not our good works. There is nothing we could ever do to make us good enough for God to save our eternal lives. Likewise, there is no way our good works could buy our success in weight loss. God's mercy toward us is the reason we are alive and free today.

Father, I thank you that you are a kind and merciful God because I know I don't deserve all you've given me. If my works determined whether or not you'd help me with weight loss and eating habits, I'd be defeated still. But you showed mercy and compassion and lifted me out of the mire as I yielded to you. Thank you, Father, in Jesus' name.

Jesus Knows Our Temptations

For in that he himself hath suffered being tempted,

145

he is able to succour them that are tempted. (Heb. 2:18)

When Jesus ascended to heaven to be with the Father, He became our high priest, but this does not mean He is so high above us that He cannot understand the things we suffer. He was once here on earth and the human part of Him suffered and was tempted just as we are. That is why He is waiting to help us when we cry for relief from our temptations.

We don't usually think that Jesus understands how much we're tempted to go into that candy store. There's a lot of suffering involved in resisting that temptation, and the enemy would have us to feel we're alone in this test; but we aren't. Just as sure as we cry to the Lord for help, Jesus is there to give us that help and relief we need.

When Jesus was out in the desert forty days and nights and faced all the enemy's temptations, He experienced every basic form of temptation and was victorious. Because of this, He is both able to sympathize with us and also show us the way out of the temptation. He is willing and able to care for us in any situation. Therefore, we should never hesitate to call on Him first. When we are confronted with that urge to cheat on our diets, let's take it straight to Jesus and receive His understanding help.

Father, thank you for sending Jesus to save me and for making Him my high priest, a high priest who understands and knows what I'm suffering. Thank you, Jesus, for always being there when I call. When that candy store is staring me in the face, I'm glad to know you're right by my side helping me to say no.

The Promise is Ours

That ye be not slothful, but followers of them who

146

through faith and patience inherit the promises. (Heb. 6:12)

We are called to walk in the same patience and faith that our forefathers from Abraham until today walked in if we are to obtain the promises of God. We cannot manipulate God; He doesn't work that way. If we are to receive from Him, we cannot be lax in our Bible study, prayer life or practical application of the biblical principles we've learned. There is no shortcut to being in God's perfect will and growing in Him.

One of the hardest things for us to learn is patient waiting for the fulfillment of God's Word to us. We diet day to day and it's often a long time before we ever see any weight loss results. This does not mean that God is failing us. He will provide in due time, but until that time our faith must stand in the place of what we've claimed for ourselves.

If we have claimed temperance as ours, we must daily continue to eat in moderation believing that one day it will be a natural part of our lives because it is God's will that we be temperate. If we continue to eat gluttonously, being impatient for God to provide temperance, it will never be ours.

The Word says we are to follow the example of those who have gone before us who through their faith in God and patience obtained the promises of God. We are the examples being set for the generation to come; therefore we must do everything according to God's Word. In this way, we show by example how the promises are fulfilled and how God is faithful to His Word.

Father, I know your Word is true and good. In the natural I'm stubborn and impatient, but by faith I can overcome these things. I will walk in your will and wait patiently for you, believing by faith that you will do even as you have said. I thank you and praise you that I know this is true.

God's Word in Your Heart

For this is the covenant that I will make with the
house of Israel after those days, saith the Lord; I will
put my laws into their mind, and write them in their
hearts: and I will be to them a God, and they shall be to
me a people. (Heb. 8:10)

God has surely fulfilled His promise in us because our hearts
convict us when we sin. First, we hear God's Word, and it is in
our heads, but we live by it only when it is rooted in our hearts.
Because of this, each of us knows God on a deep, personal
level. He is no longer way above us and difficult to reach
because He lives inside us.

If we are having trouble in any area of our lives, chances are
we do not have God's law on the subject in our hearts. Because
our hearts govern our actions, we will not walk as God would
have us if our hearts are not in line with the Word of God. It is
just as important to our spiritual lives as our physical lives that we
get the message concerning diet and eating habits into our
hearts. Therefore, we should continually be meditating on the
Word concerning this area and seeking God's will for us. It is
only then that we can take the knowledge from our heads and
place it in our hearts to live by it.

God is willing and desirous to place His Word in our hearts.
He wants us to walk in His perfect will. We can be victorious in
our dieting. We can be temperate. We can lose weight. And we
do it all through the power of God in Jesus.

Lord, I rejoice when I realize that you've placed your Word in
my heart that I might know you and live better for you. Without
the power of your Word, I could never have continued on this
diet, but your conviction is strong and I am grateful. Thank you,
Father, in Jesus' name. Continue to place more of your Word

within me that I might grow stronger in you.

Faith Includes Patience

For ye have need of patience, that, after ye have done the will of God, ye might receive the promise. (Heb. 10:36)

Paul surely must have had the dieter in mind when he was inspired to write that. Unless we patiently live daily in God's will, eating and dieting as He has told us, we will not receive the promised results. For if we are not patient, then we are anxious, and if we are anxious, then we are not moving in faith. We have already learned that without faith it is impossible to please God, and that faith is the substance from which God creates what we have claimed. Therefore, without faith, we will not receive that which we desire.

Patience in itself, however, is of no avail unless we have done the will of God and continued in that will. We cannot expect to lose weight if we consistently cheat on our diets. We cannot expect to be temperate if we insist on overeating the good foods that God has given us. We cannot hope to be free of greed if we continue to transfer our lust for bad food to lust for good food. We must be willing to yield in these areas and to walk as God directs if we hope to receive the results we desire.

It is doing God's will yesterday, today, and tomorrow in patient waiting that will bring about the weight loss and change in eating habits. Total trust in Him is His will and desire for us in all areas of our life, even eating.

Lord, patience is a hard thing for me to learn, but your Word says you won't ask me to do anything I'm not capable of doing. It's exciting just to know that this means I can be a patient person. I will follow your will and do all in patience and faith.

Discipline is for Our Good

Now no chastening for the present seemeth to be joyous, but grievous: nevertheless afterward it yieldeth the peaceable fruit of righteousness unto them which are exercised thereby. Wherefore lift up the hands which hang down, and the feeble knees. (Heb. 12:11-12)

We go around thinking we have the weight of the world on our shoulders the minute the Lord slaps our hand and says a firm no to something. We try to argue, "But, Lord, I can't live without eating sugar. It's impossible. Why are you taking it away?" The Lord just says, "Child, it's poison for your body, and you're addicted to it. It has to go if you want successful changes in your diet." So we perk up a little until God slaps something else we love out of our hands; then we're back to, "What did you do that for?"

God is not a mean Father, He's a loving one. If He corrects us and convicts us of wrong in our life, it is for our own good. No, we don't enjoy it, but we know it will bring about a change in our lives—a change which we desire very much.

So why are we still griping? We need to pick up our feet, the Word says, and quit dragging along complaining and moping. We need to get out there and work for God, use the hands and legs He gave us for Him, and forget the discomfort we're experiencing at the moment. Let us rejoice in this discipline knowing that in the end it is perfecting us and building up our strength in Him.

Father, I hate discipline, but when I realize the importance of it in my life, then I'm grateful to you for it. Remove those foods you must, Lord. Slap them out of my hand if you have to because I wish to grow closer to you in perfection each day as well as have success on my diet. Thank you for the don'ts as much as the well-dones.

For Your Perfection

My brethren, count it all joy when ye fall into diverse temptations; Knowing this, that the trying of your faith worketh patience. But let patience have her perfect work, that ye may be perfect and entire, wanting nothing. (James 1:2-4)

The last thing we want to be when temptations and tests come along is joyful. Even though we know the Bible says we should, it makes no sense to our natural minds. Our minds tell us we should complain and yell out about it, but our hearts, our spiritual parts, tell us it is all for our own good.

The Word says that when temptations come upon us, we are not only supposed to be joyful about it, but we're to be patient in it. We are not to seek to be quickly rescued from a test, but are to let our patience have a chance to fully blossom and be strengthened and perfected in us. We hate pain, especially where food is concerned, and we tend to fight patience because we're used to giving our stomachs what they want as soon as they cry out. We must learn to say no to them. Be firm in that resolve and allow patience to grow and mature inside. In this way, the Word says, we become perfected and not lacking in those good, spiritual things. Let us grow perfect in Him, for His sake, and be proved strong, faithful children of the King.

Father, I know patience is one virtue I really need an abundance of in my life. When I begin to be impatient for you to take me through a trial, remind me this trial is a good thing for me and that you are faithful to help me through in due time.

Perfect that patience within me that I might grow stronger in your image and example.

Don't Entertain Temptation

Let no man say when he is tempted, I am tempted of God: for God cannot be tempted with evil, neither tempteth He any man: But every man is tempted when he is drawn away of his own lust, and enticed. (James 1:13-14)

Passing the buck is one of our favorite tricks. We blame God for "making us this way," we blame friends for feeding us this way, we blame the devil for making us do it. The hardest part of our yielding to God was admitting that, for the most part, it was our own fault. As for the other excuses: Yes, a friend or the devil might put the thought or even the tempting food right there in front of us, but we are the ones who choose to eat it; we allow the temptation to overcome us.

When the thought of eating a whole dozen of doughnuts came to our minds, what did we do? Did we immediately throw the thought out or did we allow it to entice us to more thoughts until we gave in to lust? We all know the answer to the latter is yes.

Just because God has healed us of obesity and set us free doesn't mean we are not susceptible to temptation. Unless we are aware of how to deal with temptations when they come, we are just as likely to be carried away again and blame someone else for it. We must stand firm and say no to our fleshly lust, no to being enticed into eating as we shouldn't. When we are conscious of this fact, the battle becomes much easier to wage and victory much sweeter.

Father, I know that I am responsible for my eating habits. Keep me mindful that just because a temptation presents itself doesn't mean I have to entertain that thought or continue to look at the object tempting me. I can say no right away and avoid a difficult battle or failure.

Action, Not Words

For if any be a hearer of the word, and not a doer, he is like unto a man beholding his natural face in a glass: For he beholdeth himself, and goeth his way, and straightway forgetteth what manner of man he was. (James 1:23-24)

If there's one thing we do well, it's talk a good diet. Most of us have been on every diet that ever existed and we surely can tell you how to lose weight. So, if we knew all of that, why were we still fat? Because knowing it in our heads and knowing it in our hearts and doing it are two different things. Book knowledge in our heads, even Bible knowledge, isn't good for anything but rhetoric. It will never make a meaningful change in our lives because it does not bring about action on that knowledge.

When we heard God's Word concerning Christian weight control and eating habits, at first we couldn't accept it. Then one day we decided it was true and went around sharing it with others as if it were a new fad diet we had found. But when it came to living it, we failed as always because we had not put into our hearts (and thereby into practice) what we had learned. It was only when the conviction came deep inside and we knew for real what God's Word had to say, that we began to live it and see the life-changing results in our lives.

For years we looked in the mirror every morning, saw a fat slob and then went about eating as we pleased, forgetting how gross we already looked. Now we see ourselves as we are changing for the better and we carry that image with us, remembering to act on God's Word and not just talk about it. We achieve success now because God's Word is deep within and we are living by it, not just talking about it.

Father, thank you for planting your Word deep in my heart. I know I was a lot of talk and no action before, but thanks to your miracle in my life, I can live out my faith in you. Thank you, Lord, for setting me free deep within and guiding me daily. Keep me working and living what I believe.

Share Your Failures

Confess your faults one to another, and pray for one another, that ye may be healed. The effectual fervent prayer of a righteous man availeth much. (James 5:16)

There's nothing more detrimental to spiritual growth than hiding a mistake. If we cheat, we need to confess that sin to God, of course, but we should also acknowledge it before our brothers and sisters. Why? Well, to solicit prayer for strength and to ensure that we do not fall back into the mistake of hiding food and sneaking things behind everyone's back. It is good for us to admit out loud to others that we sin because then we can receive prayer support and put a stop to any trend toward hiding our actions.

If we are doing fine on our diets, we need to be supportive of those around us. If someone confesses a failure to us, we need to be willing and able prayer partners. What does able mean? It means we ourselves are to be righteous and in good standing with God because the Word says when we are, our prayers are powerful. Let's get in the habit of praying for each other (for healing, strength, whatever we need) and confessing our faults to each other that we might be strong.

Lord, show me when I sin (as I know you are faithful to do) that I might confess, repent, and receive forgiveness. Keep me mindful of the fact that I must not be secretive about my eating mistakes but should seek the help of a believer in prayer and discussion. Keep me close to you and ready to minister to others when they need my prayer support.

A Gradual Process

As newborn babes, desire the sincere milk of the word, that ye may grow thereby: If so be ye have tasted that the Lord is gracious. (1 Pet. 2:2-3)

When we are babies, we live on milk because it is easily digested. Without it, we could not grow stronger. God's Word is this way also; we must learn to feed on the basic simple facts first until we grow strong enough in our understanding to accept deeper truths.

Many of us see this principle in our spiritual lives in the area of diet and eating habits. God does not take away all the wrong foods at once and tell us to eat right or else! He knows we are babes in this thing and must be milk-fed, so He shows us one or two items at a time. As we receive and understand this, He makes clear less obvious errors in our diet and continues to help mature us in this way.

We are not expected to learn it all overnight, but we are also not expected to be babies all our lives. We must learn to be nourished by the Word as it is revealed to us so that we can grow into a deeper understanding of God's will. We must continue to seek God's will and His teaching on weight control and allow Him to feed us both physically and spiritually.

God is gracious. He will be gentle but firm with us, and we must understand this. We must not continue to beg for milk when He has put meat before us. As a perfect Father, He knows what and how much we can handle.

Father, I've tasted the milk of your Word, and it is good, but I know that I must be prepared for stronger food. Be firm with me and show me where I need to grow and what items still need illumination in my life. I don't want to be a baby in this area all my life because there is so much more to be done for you. Help me to grow, Lord.

Exercise Your Spirit

And beside this, giving all diligence, add to your faith virtue: and to virtue knowledge; And to knowledge temperance; and to temperance patience; and to patience godliness; And to godliness brotherly kindness; and to brotherly kindness charity. For if these things be in you, and abound, they make you that ye shall neither be barren nor unfruitful in the knowledge of our Lord Jesus Christ. (2 Pet. 1:5-8)

If we want to build up muscles in our bodies, we exercise. The more we exercise, the stronger the muscles. If we fail to exercise for a while, our muscles become weak and flabby. Well, our spiritual life is that way also. Unless we exercise the muscle of faith, we cannot hope to grow strong in our Christian walk. Each exercising we do increases and broadens our growth. Until we exercise our God-given knowledge, we will not grow in self-control or temperance. Many of us have spent years with a weak temperance muscle, but now we're beginning to get it back into the shape it should be. The more we exercise temperance, the more we also grow in patience. All of these things are interrelated. We must continue to grow and broaden our exercise program if we wish to be strong in spiritual things.

A well-exercised body finds physical exertion easier than one which is out of shape. A body that does not have good muscle tone is handicapped. When we fail to tone up our spiritual muscles, we, too, are not as efficient in working for the Lord and walking in His will.

We cannot expect physical or spiritual results to come the easy way or instantaneously. There are no shortcuts to weight loss and muscle toning; diet and exercise are the only way. Our spiritual lives are this way also. Unless we feed on a steady diet of God's Word and use what we've learned, exercising temperance, patience, and faith, we cannot hope for a strong, fruitful spiritual life.

Father, not only does my body need exercise, but my spiritual life does too. A trim, firm body isn't much use if I have a limp, malnourished spirit. Keep me going forward and using those gifts you've given me that I might grow stronger in the things of God.

Don't Return to the Pigpen

> But it is happened unto them according to the true proverb, The dog is turned to his own vomit again; and the sow that was washed to her wallowing in the mire. (2 Pet. 2:22)

We were once pigs living in gluttony and torment. If we've truly accepted our deliverance, then our lives are changed and we replace our piggishness with temperance and discipline. However, sometimes we think we've accepted the new way of life (or we try to make others believe we have) when we've only made some outward changes.

God has pulled us out of the mire, washed us clean, and there's no need to go back. If, however, the change has not occurred within, we wander back into the pigpen of greed and gluttony and get all muddied up again.

It is interesting that part of the proverb mentions a dog going back to his vomit because that is, in essence, what we do when we go back to eating as we used to. Knowing what we've done, many times we actually reach the point of vomiting because our stomachs and our consciences become sick.

Let's make that change for the Lord totally, inside as well as out, not only giving the appearance of a life change but having that change come from our inside out. There's no need to end up defeated and disgusted with ourselves. When He sets us free we can accept it, get clean, get right, and live in Him.

Lord, I never liked life in that pigpen anyway, and you certainly have lifted me out of it. I accept the totality of my freedom, inside and out.

No Self-Condemnation, Please

If we confess our sins, he is faithful and just to forgive us our sins, and to cleanse us from all unrighteousness. (1 John 1:9)

My little children, these things write I unto you, that ye sin not. And if any man sin, we have an advocate with the Father, Jesus Christ the righteous: And he is the propitiation for our sins: and not for ours only, but also for the sins of the world. And hereby we do know that we know him, if we keep his commandments. (1 John 2:1-3)

These two Scriptures tie together one central thought. We do sin. The Word says that we're liars if we say we don't. We know that if we do sin, Jesus is there, and He is the atoning sacrifice for our sins. Therefore, we know that through our confession and repentance Jesus restores our fellowship with God.

There will come times when we will feel as if we've really

blown it. For instance, blowing our dieting commitment to God for the fourth time in one week. The devil will try to tell us we've really blown it and are rotten through and through—certainly of no use to God. He knows if He can keep us thinking this way, we'll never go before the Lord in confession and our spiritual lives will be in turmoil. We must be aware of this and not fall for his trap.

The best way of avoiding this situation is to continue to study God's Word, putting it in our hearts so that we will obey His law and avoid sin. But we are told if we do sin, God will forgive us because of Jesus' blood. Therefore, we need not live in self-condemnation but must forgive ourselves even as God forgives us. This does not give us a license to sin, nor is it meant to promote a sin-now-repent-later philosophy. Anyone with this attitude surely does not love the Lord. No, it is only meant to assure us we can be forgiven and go on. Let us be quick to seek forgiveness when we sin, then seek to avoid sinning in that area again.

Lord, sometimes it's more difficult for me to forgive myself than it is for me to realize you will forgive me if I confess my sin. Your mercy is so encompassing that I can hardly understand it. Thank you, Lord, for sending Jesus to not only make forgiveness possible but to show me how to live so that I could avoid sin. Keep me in your perfect will and warn me when I step out of it.

As Jesus Walked

He that saith he abideth in him ought himself also so to walk, even as he walked. (1 John 2:6)

For years we've said we're walking with the Lord and abiding in the vine, but our very appearance and habits said that was all a lie. We were no more abiding in Him than the heathens. Why? Because we were not walking as He walked, as we are called to walk. We lived in gluttony, greed, obesity, depression, and defeat. This certainly does not describe the walk Jesus walked.

When we heard about Christian weight control, we were excited because we could foresee the freedom and good health (as well as slim bodies) it could provide. But did we consider that we should have been eating and living that way all the time because it is part of walking as Jesus did? Did we realize temperance is for the skinny as well as the fat, the healthy as well as the unhealthy?

We need to learn to judge every thought, action, and deed according to the standards that Jesus set. If it is not in line with what Jesus would have done, we shouldn't be doing it. For instance, Jesus didn't live in sickness. Since obesity is a disease, we should have no part of it. It is not a Christ-like way to live. Greed, gluttony, compulsive eating are all contrary to the will of God and the way in which Jesus walked, and should not be a part of our lives either. Jesus lived in victory; so should we. In all things we must abide in Him and live even as He did. It is important that we become slim and healthy. It is more important that we make our lives conform to the example set by Jesus simply because we love Him and desire to live for Him and please Him.

Lord, keep me ever mindful that my thoughts and actions must be in line with the Word. If I am to become like Jesus, I must walk in the same way in which He walked. Gluttony, greed, fatness—those are not Christ-like, and I will not have them as part of my life. Help me to grow and mature in my walk, Lord.

Greater is the Spirit Within

Ye are of God, little children, and have overcome them; because greater is he that is in you, than he that is in the world. (1 John 4:4)

As Christians, we are supposed to be living our lives in victory over the devil and this world because Jesus has overcome the world. However, many of us are so used to living in defeat that we forget it doesn't have to be that way. We've been on so many diets and tried to lose weight so many times only to end up worse off than before. We've wished we could eat healthy and be satisfied with moderation, but it has not worked for us.

The Holy Spirit is here to proclaim anew and remind us that there is no need for us to lose the diet battle, because the Holy Spirit which is within us is greater than the devil. We, through the Spirit, have the powerful weapons of faith and the Word of God, and if we use these weapons to fight the enemy, we will win. We should never again confess or accept failure. We have the power of God within us and we are already more than conquerors through Christ Jesus. Let's live in that victory because we've won the battle against fat and gluttony.

Lord, I've been such a fool to think that I've lost the battle again. Forgive me, in Jesus' name, for doubting that you had the power to give me the victory. I will no longer sit in a corner feeling defeated and frustrated but will stand up and fight, knowing I have already won through the Holy Spirit, my Teacher, Comforter and Protector. Thank you, Father, in Jesus' sweet and powerful name.

Faith Overcomes

For whatsoever is born of God overcometh the world:
and this is the victory that overcometh the world, even
our faith. (1 John 5:4)

We are born of God if we have accepted Jesus as our Savior.
He died for our sins, rose from the dead, and is with the Father
serving as our high priest. If this is true, then the Word says that
we've already overcome the world by the victory wrought by
our faith. It is our belief and trust in Jesus' power to save us from
eternal damnation that brought about our salvation. That belief
had to be in our hearts and confessed with our mouths before
we actually became children of God and possessed eternal life.
Victory in other areas is achieved in the same way.

Just knowing in our heads that the Word says we've
overcome the world will never make it a functioning reality in
our lives. Knowing that God is able to set us free from fat, greed,
and gluttony doesn't take one ounce of fat off our bodies. Why?
Because we must believe in our hearts that He not only can but
will do this for us, and confess it with our mouths, thus proving
our faith in Him. At that moment, we've overcome the problem.
We cannot see it with our eyes, but our faith stands in place of
seeing the results until we can see them.

Without faith we're already defeated, but with faith in God
we've overcome the world and all of its pain and bondage. We
need never fear fat, gluttony, or greed because our faith in God
will sustain us in victory.

Lord, where would I be without you? It amazes me that I
could ever have doubted your strength and power. I know that
you are in the miracle business today and that I've overcome the
world through my faith in you and the power of the blood of
Jesus.

We Are Winners

And hath made us kings and priests unto God and his
Father; to him be glory and dominion for ever and
ever. Amen. (Rev. 1:6)

Isn't it good to come to the end of the Bible and find out that
we will be winners throughout eternity? The Word says that we
are all kings and priests through the atonement of Jesus and His
regaining dominion over the earth for us. Adam, one man, lost
dominion to the devil, but Jesus, one man, won it back again by
conquering death, hell and Satan.

Because of what Jesus has done, we can live in the peace and
assurance that victory over Satan and the world are ours
now. We are kings and priests through Him, and it is time we
started living like it.

Kings don't take orders from their subjects and neither should
we. Jesus has put Satan and his hosts under our feet, and we are
to command and rule him, not vice versa. He cannot lay fat,
gluttony, or greed on us because we don't have to take it. All we
need to take is authority over the enemy and command him to
leave in Jesus' name, and he has to go.

We are priests also and are to live our lives ministering to the
Lord (in praise and worship) and to others. All of our thoughts,
words and deeds should attain one common goal—to bring
honor and glory to our King, who is worthy of all we have to give
and more. Let us go forth into the world to live as kings and
priests of the Lord, showing forth His glory that He might
receive all honor and praise.

Sweet heavenly Father, I want my life to reflect your glory and
power. Forgive my selfishness and lust, in Jesus' name. Use me
in whatever way you desire and perfect me in body, mind, and
spirit, that all might see your infinite wisdom and power.

For free information on how to receive
the international magazine

LOGOS JOURNAL

with NATIONAL COURIER update
also Book Catalog

Write: Information - LOGOS JOURNAL CATALOG
Box 191
Plainfield, NJ 07061